Department of Veterans Affairs
Health Services Research & Development Service | Evidence-based Synthesis Program

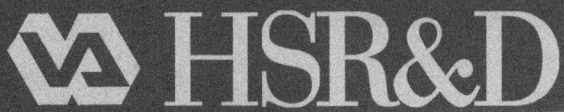

I0470836

A Systematic Evidence Review of Interventions for Non-professional Caregivers of Individuals with Dementia

October 2010

Prepared for:
Department of Veterans Affairs
Veterans Health Administration
Health Services Research & Development Service
Washington, DC 20420

Prepared by:
Evidence-based Synthesis Program (ESP) Center
Portland VA Medical Center
Portland, OR

Devan Kansagara, MD, MCR, Director

Investigators:
Principal Investigator:
Elizabeth Goy, PhD
Co-Investigator:
Devan Kansagara, MD, MCR

Research Associate:
Michele Freeman, MPH

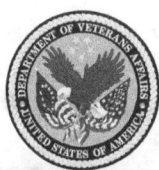

PREFACE

HSR&D's Evidence-based Synthesis Program (ESP) was established to provide timely and accurate syntheses of targeted healthcare topics of particular importance to VA managers and policymakers, as they work to improve the health and healthcare of Veterans. The ESP disseminates these reports throughout VA.

HSR&D provides funding for four ESP Centers and each Center has an active VA affiliation. The ESP Centers generate evidence syntheses on important clinical practice topics, and these reports help:

- develop clinical policies informed by evidence,
- the implementation of effective services to improve patient outcomes and to support VA clinical practice guidelines and performance measures, and
- set the direction for future research to address gaps in clinical knowledge.

In 2009, an ESP Coordinating Center was created to expand the capacity of HSR&D Central Office and the four ESP sites by developing and maintaining program processes. In addition, the Center established a Steering Committee comprised of HSR&D field-based investigators, VA Patient Care Services, Office of Quality and Performance, and VISN Clinical Management Officers. The Steering Committee provides program oversight and guides strategic planning, coordinates dissemination activities, and develops collaborations with VA leadership to identify new ESP topics of importance to Veterans and the VA healthcare system.

Comments on this evidence report are welcome and can be sent to Nicole Floyd, ESP Coordinating Center Program Manager, at nicole.floyd@va.gov.

Recommended citation:
Goy E, Freeman M, Kansagara D. A Systematic Evidence Review of Interventions for Non-professional Caregivers of Individuals with Dementia. VA-ESP Project #05-225: 2010

TABLE OF CONTENTS

EXECUTIVE SUMMARY

BACKGROUND

The purpose of this report is to review systematically the evidence on the effects of caregiver (CG) interventions on CG burden, mood (including depression and anxiety), and the ability to manage problematic behavior, as well as the effects on the care recipient (CR).

METHODS

We conducted a review of good-quality trials identified from systematic reviews and additional studies identified from expert input. We conducted searches for systematic reviews of dementia CG interventions in MEDLINE (PubMed), the Cochrane Database of Systematic Reviews, and the Cochrane Database of Reviews of Effects from database inception through July 2009.

RESULTS

There were 15 systematic reviews that met our quality criteria: one review of respite care, three reviews of technology-based interventions, and 12 systematic reviews that evaluated a variety of heterogeneous psychosocial interventions. The systematic reviews of psychosocial interventions identified 30 randomized controlled trials (RCTs) that met our criteria for study design and sample size. Seven good quality RCTs recommended by expert panel members were added following review.

KEY QUESTION #1. Do CG interventions affect the CG's knowledge and ability to manage problematic behavior, CG psychosocial burden, CG health and health behaviors, or outcomes in the individual with dementia?

PSYCHOSOCIAL INTERVENTIONS

Multicomponent Interventions: Five studies evaluated a combination of varied treatment approaches such as skills training, group support, and respite care. Three of the studies examined individually tailored multicomponent interventions. Individually tailored intensive, multicomponent interventions showed promise for reducing CG depression, and in improving sense of burden, self-care abilities, well-being, confidence, and social support ratings. When examined across diverse populations, there were group effects for all Latino/Hispanic and White/Caucasian CGs as well as Black/African-American spousal CGs. Additionally, CGs who experience individually crafted interventions during their caregiving period may fare better during the bereavement phase. There was no consistent evidence that multicomponent interventions delayed CR institutionalization.

Exercise Training: We reviewed one trial that compared exercise training for the CG with an attention-control group that received supportive phone calls and nutrition guidance. Both exercise and control groups demonstrated decreased depression, stress, and burden, but there were no significant differences between groups. More studies are needed to evaluate the impact of exercise for the CG on CG burden.

Case Management Interventions: We reviewed five studies of intensive nursing case management. Overall intensive nursing case management had little effect on CR rates of institutionalization, but improvements in CG outcomes were seen in some studies. One study reported lower rates of institutionalization for the first months of the two-year program, but by the end of two years there were no differences in rates of insitutionalization between intervention and control groups. Two other studies found no differences between case management and usual care in time to institutionalization, or in CG strain, burden, or depression. Two studies published in 2006 support that case management can result in improvements in CG stress (at 12 but not 18 months), confidence, mastery of caregiving skills, and depression (seen at 18 months). These same studies reported smaller declines for CR health related quality of life and fewer CR behavioral symptoms, although CR rates of institutionalization remained the same for treatment and control groups.

Behavior Management Training (BMT): Four studies were reviewed that provide limited evidence suggesting that training the CG to use behavioral management techniques with the CR may improve CG depression, although this finding was not consistent across all studies. Two studies in which BMT for the CG was augmented by a separate component – CG self-care instruction in one study; exercise for the CR in another – seemed to result in broader outcome effects, with reports of improved CR physical mobility and CG coping skills.

Individual Skills Training: Two of six studies demonstrated that individual skills training for CGs ameliorates depression in CGs, but the data show no support for impact on CGs' sense of burden, anxiety, or quality of life. In three studies, CRs showed slower declines in self-care when skills training included a component targeting activities of daily living (ADL), and improved mood when pleasant events were scheduled, but these findings were not replicated in three other studies. Two of six studies reported that disruptive behavior may be reduced when CGs receive structured training in identifying triggers of disruptive behavior and modifying the environment to reduce stress. There is no strong evidence documenting the impact of skills training programs on delaying or preventing institutionalization of the CR.

Group Skills Training Interventions: CG depression improved in three of eight intervention studies; significant effects may be associated with interventions that are individualized by in-home assessment and targeted to specific needs of the CR-CG dyad. Two studies reported reductions in CG distress. Ancillary improvements in positive interactions and nurturing, reducing aversive and hostile CG responses to problem behaviors, reducing CG burden, and increasing CG self-efficacy are supported by single studies in the skills training domain.

Individual, Group, and Combined Individual/Group Supportive CG Counseling Interventions: In seven studies reviewed, neither individual supportive counseling nor group supportive interventions *on their own* demonstrated clear superiority over control groups for CG depression. A combined individual/group approach resulted in delayed institutionalization for the CR and improved mood for the CG, with results sustained across three years in follow-up. Ancillary improvements in affective regulation for coping and aversive reaction to CR behavior disturbance were supported in single studies. None of these interventions demonstrated group treatment effects for CG burden.

TECHNOLOGY-BASED INTERVENTIONS

Three systematic reviews assessed the effectiveness of networked information and communications technology interventions (ICT). These included five interventions that used computer-telephone integrated support systems, and 13 interventions that aimed to increase patient safety and reduce CG stress, such as Global Positioning System (GPS) location systems and home-monitoring devices (e.g., boundary alarms, cooking monitors). The evidence from controlled empirical studies on the effectiveness of technology-based interventions is insufficient, but uncontrolled studies suggest that GPS location systems for wandering behavior may improve patient function and safety, as well as reduce CG depression, burden, and stress. Robust trials with sufficient follow-up are needed to determine the feasibility, effectiveness, and cost-effectiveness of ICT interventions.

RESPITE CARE

A comprehensive systematic review of the effectiveness and cost-effectiveness of respite care services was compiled in 2004 for the United Kingdom (UK) National Health Service (NHS). The review identified 45 studies on several forms of respite care, and found small, statistically-significant improvements on some outcome measures, but the evidence on how respite affects the health and well-being of CGs was inconsistent. Institutional/overnight respite promoted better sleep patterns in CGs during the period of respite; but there were no enduring improvements in health and well-being in comparison to control groups, or compared to CG baseline state associated with respite services of any form. The vast majority of CGs, however, frequently expressed high levels of satisfaction, and generally felt that respite services brought them various benefits, despite little evidence of significant and/or sustained reductions in measures of stress, depression, and burden. Many studies reported CGs' beliefs that respite enabled them to continue caregiving.

RECENT AND ONGOING VA STUDIES

A recently completed six-month implementation study of the Resources for Enhancing Alzheimer's Caregiver Health (REACH) Veterans Affairs (VA) intervention found positive effects on CG burden and CR problem behaviors, and appears to be feasible in VA settings. The multicomponent intervention includes CG support and skills training in safety, behavior management, and self care via in-home, telephone, and telephone support group sessions. Other CG interventions recently or currently being studied in VA include the Telehealth Education Program (a telephone-based education and support group); Telephone-Linked Care (TLC, a computer-mediated telephone support system); Partners in Dementia Care (PDC), a collaborative intervention delivered by care coordinators from local VA Medical Centers (VAMCs) and Alzheimer's Association chapters; and the use of remote sensor technology to monitor Veterans in the Home-based Primary Care program.

Key Question #2. What are adverse effects of CG interventions?

The systematic review of respite care found evidence in one study to suggest that CGS using day care service actually spend more time on caregiving activities on respite days than on non-respite days, usually in preparing the CR for the visit or transporting the CR to the day care setting. In a small study of institutional/overnight respite services, some CGs reported feelings of sadness, loneliness, or guilt while the CR was in respite care; and some reported criticism from friends and relatives for allowing relief admission. A drawback of overnight respite care reported by some CGs was that the disruption to the CR's routine had increased the patient's anxiety and confusion, and that there was an increase in short-term workload on return home.

We found no evidence of adverse effects from other CG interventions based on the systematic reviews yielded by our search, and the primary studies on psychosocial interventions we examined.

DISCUSSION

CG interventions that appear to be effective tend to be individually-tailored treatments that are more resource-intensive, such as BMT, multicomponent interventions, and individual skills training. Overall, the strongest support appears for multicomponent interventions that are designed after individual in-home assessment, and tailored to the specific needs of the CG/CR dyad. The feasibility of implementation and cost analyses of CG interventions need to be assessed within VA settings. Individualized programs may be the most effective but would require more resources of staff to evaluate the dyad and generate a tailored program.

Loss to follow-up appeared problematic for many of the studies in this review, and may be clinically important. This may highlight issues of intervention acceptability to dementia CGs, and reasons for dropout should be assessed and help guide future implementation efforts in this field.

Respite care may offer some short term benefits to CGs though long-term benefits have not been shown. Health services research evaluating cost effectiveness of variations of this intervention within the VA setting may help identify the most beneficial length for respite and contribute to policy decisions regarding this intervention.

The wide range of outcomes used to evaluate the effects of CG interventions reflects the diversity in what CGs and researchers consider important. Qualitative studies to identify outcomes of supportive interventions that are important to individuals with dementia and their CGs within the VA system would serve future research and policy for promoting the best welfare of aging Veterans and their community CGs.

INTRODUCTION

BACKGROUND

In 2004, the Office of the Assistant Deputy Under Secretary for Health for Policy and Planning estimated that the total number of Veterans with dementia would be as high as 563,758 in FY 2010.[1] Individuals with dementia are frequently cared for at home by a friend or family member. The progressive nature of the illness and the intensity of care that may be required in caring for a loved one with dementia have physical, emotional, and psychological impacts on the CG. The purpose of this report is to review systematically the evidence on the effects of CG interventions on CG burden, mood (including depression and anxiety), and ability to manage problematic behavior, as well as the effects on the CR.

The Veterans Health Administration (VHA) Office of Geriatrics and Extended Care (OGEC) in Patient Care Services has primary responsibility for coordination and direction of VHA dementia initiatives. OGEC convened an interdisciplinary Dementia Steering Committee (DSC) in December 2006, with the goal of making recommendations on comprehensive, coordinated care for Veterans with dementia. The DSC requested VA Health Services Research and Development's (HSR&D) Evidence-based Synthesis Program (ESP) to review evidence on selected topics, in order to assist with DSC planning efforts. The DSC served as the technical expert panel for guiding topic development and reviewing drafts of the report.

METHODS

TOPIC DEVELOPMENT

The review was requested by the VHA DSC, and the DSC served as the technical expert panel for guiding topic development and reviewing drafts of the report.

The objectives of this review are to address the following questions:

Key Question #1: Do CG interventions affect the CG's knowledge and ability to manage problematic behavior, psychosocial burden, health and health behaviors, or outcomes in the individual with dementia?

Key Question #2: What are adverse effects of CG interventions?

Population: Non-professional CGs of individuals with dementia in all settings. CGs include spouses and other family members, as well as paid sitters or assistants hired by the family; professional staff is excluded.

Interventions: Categories of intervention include psychoeducational interventions, cognitive-behavioral interventions, counseling/case management, general support services, respite care, and multicomponent interventions. Specific interventions of interest targeted CGs and included telephone-based support groups and education, Home TeleHealth/Health Buddy home monitoring device; Internet-based resources and CG assistance programs, and physical activity.

Comparator: Usual care / no interventions directed at the CG.

CG outcomes:

- Knowledge and ability to manage problematic behavior;
- Psychosocial outcomes (burden/subjective well-being, depression, anxiety, perceived self-efficacy, positive experiences of caregiving, satisfaction with health care, quality of life);
- Health behaviors (diet, exercise, sleep);
- Health (reported health, symptoms, medication use/misuse, service use, mortality).

CR outcomes:

- Use of psychotropic drugs;
- Cognition, mood, behavioral disturbances, social function, or physical function;
- Hospitalizations, institutionalizations, or health care visits including ER visits;
- Accidents;
- Health-related quality of life;
- Satisfaction with health care.

Setting: Home, community living center.

The DSC served as the technical expert panel for guiding topic development and reviewing drafts of the report.

SEARCH STRATEGY

We conducted a search for systematic reviews of dementia CG interventions in MEDLINE (PubMed), using the following search terms: ("dementia"[MeSH Terms] OR "dementia"[All Fields]) AND systematic[sb]. We also searched in the Cochrane Database of Systematic Reviews and the Cochrane Database of Reviews of Effects (OVID) from database inception through July 2009, using the term dementia.mp. In addition to the search for published systematic reviews, we contacted researchers within VA to identify important recent and ongoing studies of dementia CG interventions. We also examined recently published studies found in a compendium compiled by the Administration on Aging's (AoA) Alzheimer's Disease Supportive Services Program[2] that were not captured in previous systematic reviews. All citations were imported into an electronic database (EndNote X2).

STUDY SELECTION

Three reviewers assessed the titles and abstracts of citations identified from literature searches. Full-text articles of potentially relevant abstracts were retrieved for further review. We selected systematic reviews of CG interventions, using the eligibility criteria shown in Appendix A. Eligible articles had English-language abstracts and provided data relevant to the key questions.

Eligibility criteria varied depending on the question of interest, as described below.

The literature search identified four systematic reviews that focused on respite care, and six reviews on technology-based interventions. We selected one systematic review on respite care and three reviews on technology-based interventions that were the most comprehensive, recent, and relevant.

There were 10 systematic reviews that evaluated a variety of psychosocial interventions, including exercise, case management, behavioral management training, individual and group skills training, individual support or counseling, and multicomponent interventions. We examined the degree of overlap between articles included in systematic reviews and found that many of the primary studies were included in more than one review. We also found that the systematic reviews grouped psychosocial interventions in different ways, combining a variety of dissimilar therapies in some cases. This made it difficult to summarize the findings of previous systematic reviews on the effects of specific forms of treatment. We therefore retrieved the full-text articles for the primary studies included in these systematic reviews, and examined each study for quality (see Quality Assessment section below), design, and type of intervention. Out of concern that we might miss content from good quality primary studies that were reviewed elsewhere (in systematic reviews excluded from our sample due to poor quality), we retained one very comprehensive systematic review[3] that had identified 127 CG intervention studies but did not meet our quality criteria for systematic reviews. This effort contributed an additional three RCTs to our review of primary data on psychosocial interventions.

Altogether there were 224 primary studies included among the 11 systematic reviews of psychosocial interventions. Of these, we selected RCTs rated good-quality by the respective systematic review and with sample size greater than 50, and analyzed the body of evidence for specific forms of treatment. This approach allowed us to identify the best evidence for specific psychosocial interventions, based on the literature searches and quality assessments previously conducted by existing systematic reviews.

Our expert review panel recommended additional individual studies published after the search dates of the respective systematic reviews, and were considered by panel members to demonstrate important advances in the field. We also examined studies found in the compendium of intervention studies compiled by the AoA Alzheimer's Disease Supportive Services Program. These studies met our criteria for inclusion as good quality, RCTs, and were incorporated into our overall review.

DATA ABSTRACTION

For technology-based interventions and respite care, we summarized the findings of recent systematic reviews that had performed comprehensive, qualitative syntheses of the primary literature on these topics.

From RCTs on psychosocial interventions, we abstracted information about sample characteristics; the methods used for the intervention and control groups; the outcome measures used; and the results for CG and CR. We compiled evidence tables organized for the psychosocial interventions.

QUALITY ASSESSMENT

We rated the quality of systematic reviews using the criteria shown in Appendix B.[4, 5] We selected good-quality systematic reviews based on the comprehensiveness and reproducibility of the search strategy, the use of standard methods to appraise the validity of included studies, and the absence of apparent bias in drawing conclusions.

As noted, we also included one systematic review[3] that did not meet our quality criteria (the methods for quality rating were not reproducible as described), because it included the most comprehensive report of primary studies, and improved our confidence that we were not missing good quality primary studies. We examined 78 controlled trials of psychosocial interventions that had been previously rated high in quality by existing systematic reviews, by considering the following elements: the comparability of treatment groups; the adequacy of randomization; whether treatment allocation was concealed; whether eligibility criteria were specified; the use of blinding among patients, care providers, and outcome assessors; whether the analysis was intention-to-treat, or conducted with post-randomization exclusions, or with extensive or differential loss to follow-up; clearly defined interventions; and reliable outcome measurement (Appendix C).[4] We applied criteria for randomization and adequate sample size (n≥50) to select uniformly the studies that would most likely represent the best evidence on a particular intervention, among the controlled trials that had been identified and screened by good quality systematic reviews.

DATA SYNTHESIS

We organized the literature into the following intervention categories:

- Psychosocial interventions
  - o Multicomponent interventions
  - o Exercise training
  - o Case management
  - o Behavioral management training
  - o Individual skills training
  - o Group skills training
  - o Individual, group, and combined individual/group supportive counseling
- Technology-based interventions
- Respite care

We selected systematic reviews on respite care and technology-based interventions that had performed recent, thorough assessments of the relevant evidence, and therefore represent the current knowledge available on these topics. We chose to present a summary of their findings directly in this report. For psychosocial interventions, which were far more heterogeneous, we critically analyzed primary trials selected to represent the best evidence on these topics according to the criteria listed above. We compiled a qualitative, descriptive synthesis of the evidence on specific forms of therapy: exercise, case management, behavioral management training, individual and group skills training, individual support or counseling, and multicomponent interventions.

A list of abbreviations is provided in Appendix D.

PEER REVIEW

A draft version of this report was sent to the technical advisory panel and additional peer reviewers. Their comments and our responses resulted in updates to our review and are included in Appendix E.

RESULTS

LITERATURE SEARCH

Figure 1 shows the yield and flow of the literature search. The search for systematic reviews yielded 1,711 citations. After abstract review (see Appendix A), de-duplication of remaining articles retrieved from both databases, and the removal of systematic reviews that had been updated (for example, if there were three Cochrane reviews on a topic, only the most recent update was retained), a total of 112 review articles were retained for full-text review. Of these, we included 15 that met our criteria for good quality systematic reviews (Appendix B). We included one review of respite care and three reviews of technology-based interventions.

There were 11 systematic reviews that evaluated a variety of psychosocial interventions in 224 primary studies. Of these, we examined 78 primary studies that had been rated good quality in the systematic reviews. Among these 78 studies, we identified 30 RCTs of psychosocial interventions that met our quality criteria for study design and sample size.

We also examined three good-quality studies found in the compendium of intervention studies compiled by the AoA Alzheimer's Disease Supportive Services Program,[2] six studies that were identified by peer reviewers, and one good quality RCT published just as we were concluding our response to peer review.

Figure 1. Literature Flow

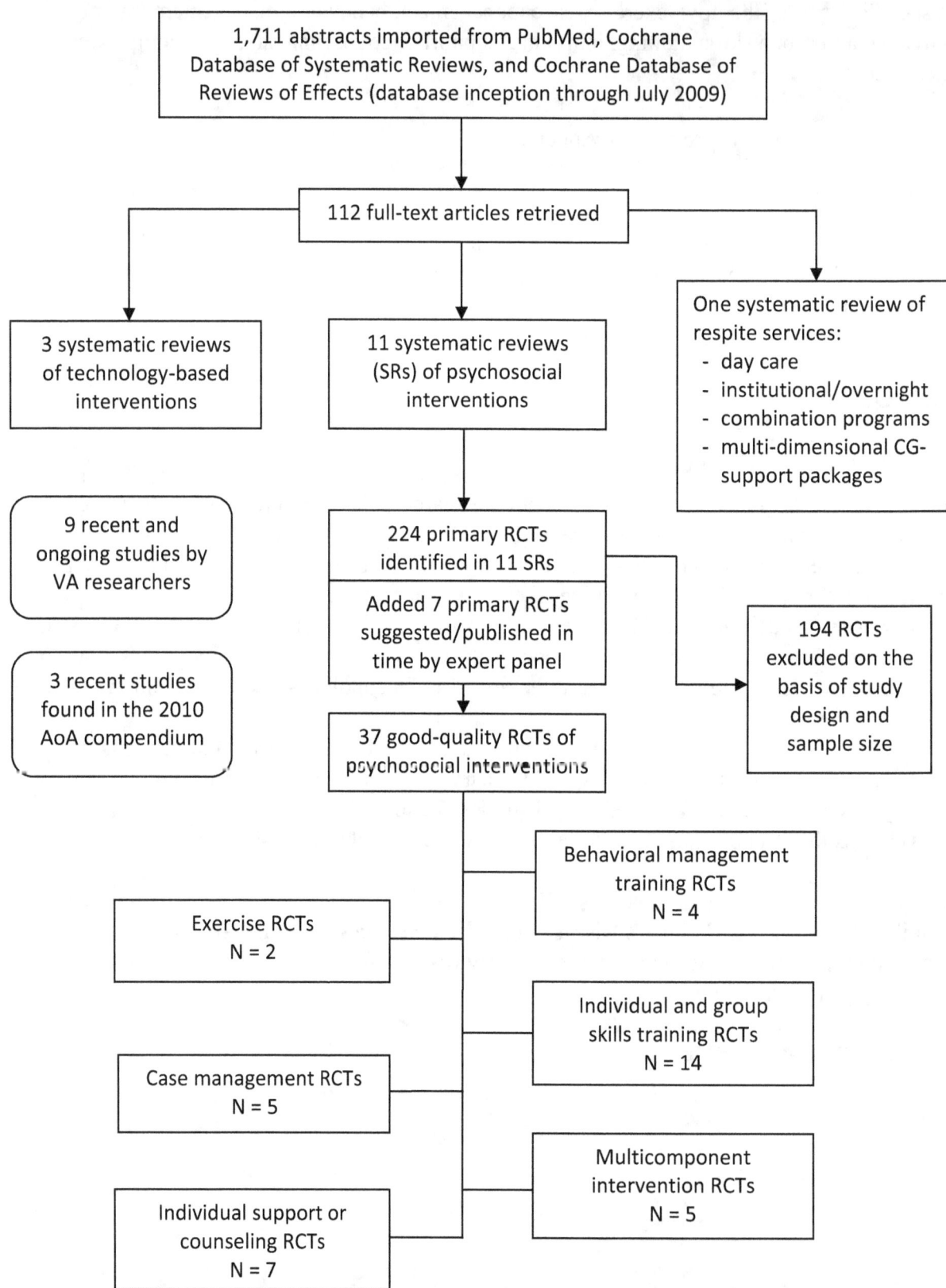

KEY QUESTION #1. Do CG interventions affect the CG's knowledge and ability to manage problematic behavior, psychosocial burden, health and health behaviors, or outcomes in the individual with dementia?

PSYCHOSOCIAL INTERVENTIONS

The results on psychosocial interventions are organized in the following subcategories: multicomponent studies; exercise training; case management; behavior management training (BMT); individual skills training; group skills training and combined individual/group skills training; and individual, group, and combined individual/group supportive counseling.

MULTICOMPONENT STUDIES

Summary impact of multicomponent interventions: There is no consistent evidence that multicomponent interventions delayed CR institutionalization. Individually tailored intensive, multicomponent interventions show promise for reducing CG depression, and in improving sense of burden, self care abilities, well-being, confidence, and social support ratings. When examined across diverse populations, there were group effects for all Latino/Hispanic and White/Caucasian CGs, as well as Black/African-American spousal CGs. Additionally, CGs who experience individually crafted interventions during their caregiving period may fare better during the bereavement phase.

Five studies evaluated a combination of varied treatment approaches such as skills training, group support, and respite care (Table 1). In one study, two treatment groups were compared to a respite control condition.[6] CGs in Treatment 1 received 10 days of structured group support and skills training to improve coping, set limits, seek support, reduce guilt, and reframe challenges while living in a residential setting (as non-admissions in a psychiatric ward of a general teaching hospital) while CRs participated in separate structured training for memory enhancement. Follow-up phone calls and trainings continued for 12 months. Treatment 2 consisted of a six-month wait list, then entry into similar treatment and follow-up for 12 months. Both groups were compared to a control condition in which the CG received 10 days respite with phone follow-up similar to Treatment 1. All CRs across the three conditions received 10-day memory activity training. CRs of CGs who received training (Treatments 1 & 2 combined) had significantly delayed institutionalization compared to respite control, with effects evident across eight years in survival analysis. No other outcomes were reported. The three groups were comparable for average age of CGs and CRs, CR performance on the Mini Mental Status Examination,[7] average CR performance on the Clinical Dementia Rating Scale,[8] and rates of decline on measures of instrumental ADL and ADL at 3, 6, and 12 months after training.

The second study provided weekly in-home respite care (four hours) plus weekly home visits by a nurse to provide CG education and training, and monthly self-help CG support groups for six months.[9] This intervention was compared to usual care control offering community nursing focused on the CR rather than CG, with monitoring of medicines and help with activities of living. While the intervention was associated with a favorable cost per quality-adjusted life year gained, no significant differences in CG or CR depression, anxiety, quality of life, or time to institutionalization were reported.

We considered two studies completed after the previous systematic reviews were published, on the recommendation of our expert panel. An RCT compared a six-month individually tailored program of 12 in-home and telephone interventions (including skills training, problem solving, stress management training, and five structured phone support group sessions with supplemental written resource materials) with control participants who received written informational materials plus an invitation to join a group at the end of data collection (N =642).[10] This study also examined the impact of the intervention for different ethnicities, including Hispanic/Latino (N = 212), Black/African-American (N = 211), and White/Caucasian (N = 219). The overall prevalence of CG depression was higher in the control group at follow-up. Hispanic and White participants endorsed significant improvements for depression, burden, self-care, and social support (referred to collectively as "quality of life"), but in the Black group, these findings were supported for spousal CGs only. Clinical improvement (defined as change equal to or greater than 0.5 Standard Deviation) across all measured domains was greater for the CG intervention group than the control group for Hispanic/Latino participants. White CG participants demonstrated clinically meaningful improvements in social support. Black CG participants showed clinically meaningful differences for burden and self care, for spouses only. White and Hispanic CRs had significantly greater improvements in problem behaviors following treatment when compared to control members, but this change did not occur among Black CRs. The intervention had no effect on institutionalization at follow-up.

The second of these recent studies comprised a subset (N = 224) of the REACH program of research, reporting the impact of various REACH interventions and their paired controls across the country on postmortem grief experiences of dementia CGs.[11] Overall, CGs who participated in the intervention groups prior to the death of their CR endorsed less normal grief than in the control conditions. There was a nonsignificant trend for reduced complicated grief in the intervention group. No group treatment effects were seen for CG depression. The authors observed across REACH sites that cognitive-behavioral interventions appeared most effective in preventing complicated grief.

A fifth good quality RCT[12] was released for publication during our response to peer review. Originating with the Care of Persons with Dementia in their Environments (COPE) trial, this study conducted individual home assessment (N = 102) of CR deficits and CG concerns, followed by up to 12 home or telephone visits over four months providing: CG education about their partner's capabilities, medications, and symptoms; and CG training to address problem behaviors, improve communication, simplify tasks, and reduce environmental stressors, compared to a control group (N = 107) receiving three phone calls and educational materials. Intervention participants demonstrated better outcomes than the control group for CR instrumental ADL and overall functional dependence, CR activity engagement, and CG wellbeing and reported confidence. These effects were still apparent at nine-month follow-up for CGs, but not for CRs.

Limitations of the literature: In the initial studies reviewed, group sizes were small, ranging from 30-33 across both studies, possibly limiting power to detect change. One study found a treatment effect on time to CR institutionalization, but it is difficult to ascertain which aspect(s) of the multicomponent treatment were effective in these studies.

Table 1. RCTs of multicomponent interventions for caregivers of individuals with dementia

Study	Brodaty, et al. 1997[6]	Drummond, et al. 1991[9]	Belle, et al. 2006[10] REACH II	Holland, et al. 2009[11]	Gitlin, et al. 2010[12]
Population (N)	Individuals with dementia and their coresident CG. (N=96, with 93 completing)	CG living with a cognitively impaired relative judged unlikely to be institutionalized during study. (N=60)	Individuals with AD or related disorders and their caregivers who reported distress associated with caregiving, grouped by caregiver ethnicity. (Hispanic/Latino N = 212, White/Caucasian N = 219, Black/African-American N = 211). (642)	Bereaved family caregivers of decedent individuals who had Alzheimer's dementia. (N = 224, subset of REACH study)	Individuals with dementia and their family CGs who reported difficulty managing CR functional decline or behaviors. (N=209)
Intervention (N)	All CRs received 10-day training on memory tips and activities. Treatment 1) CG received 10-day structured residential training to improve coping, set limits, seek support, reduce guilt, and reframe challenges, with follow-up phone calls and trainings for 12 mos. (N=33) Treatment 2) Wait list, entered into treatment 1 after waiting 6 months, similar follow-up for 6 mos. (N=31)	Weekly in-home respite care (4 hours), weekly nurse home visits to provide education and training, and monthly self-help support group for 6 months. (N=30)	Six month program of 12 in-home and telephone individually tailored active interventions including skills training, problem solving, stress management training, and didactics, with 5 structured phone support group sessions. Written resource materials supplemented training. (N =323; 106, 113, 104, respectively by ethnicity)	Active interventions varied across REACH sites, often multicomponent, included behavioral interventions, environmental modifications, support directly and/or by phone and/or computer	Tailored assessment, CG education, CG training. 102 dyads received up to 10 sessions with an occupational therapist over 4 months, and 1 face-to-face session and 1 phone session with an advance practice nurse.
Control (N)	CG received 10 days respite with similar follow-up to Tx1. (N=30)	Usual care community nursing focused on the CR rather than CG, monitoring medicines and helping with ADL/IADLs. (N=30)	Mailed educational packet, 2 brief phone contacts, plus invitation to join dementia/caregiving workshop at the end of the study (N = 319; 106, 106, 107 respectively)	Varied across sites, included minimal support and usual care conditions.	Controlled for professional attention and tailoring of information. 107 dyads received up to 3 20-minute phone calls from research staff (not occupational therapists or nurses), and general information brochures.
CG outcome measures	Not evaluated	CQLI CES-D STAI	CES-D, Zarit Caregiver Burden Interview, 11-item health self-care questions 10 items social support measure	Inventory of Complicated Grief Texas Revised Inventory of Grief CES=D	Well-being: 13-item perceived change index (ability to manage dementia, emotional status, somatic symptoms); Confidence: 5-item activities in last month; Satisfaction, perceived benefits.

Study	Brodaty, et al. 1997[6]	Drummond, et al. 1991[9]	Belle, et al. 2006[10] REACH II	Holland, et al. 2009[11]	Gitlin, et al. 2010[12]
CG results	Not evaluated.	No significant differences in depression, anxiety, or quality of life.	Significantly greater (statistical) improvements among Hispanic/Latino and White/Cauc participants for depression, burden, self-care, social support, but not for Black/AA participants. Black/AA spouses showed significantly greater improvement than spouses in control group (but not nonspouses). Net clinical improvement across 5 domains greater in intervention than control group for Hispanic/Latino participants. White participants showed clinically meaningful effect with social support. Black/AA participants showed clinically meaningful differences for burden and self care, for spouses only. Overall prevalence of depression higher for controls at follow-up.	CGs in intervention groups reported significantly fewer normal grief symptoms than control condition. Nonsignificant trend for reduced complicated grief in intervention group. No effects seen for depression. Cognitive-behavioral interventions seem to be most effective as preventative for complicated grief.	Adjusted mean difference (95% CI) at 4 months: Improved well-being, PCI: 0.22 (0.08-0.36) Confidence using activities: 0.81 (0.30-1.32) More COPE CGs reported eliminating at least 1 problem: 62.7% vs. 44.9% (p=0.01).
CR outcome measures	ADL IADL Months to nursing home admission Months to death	Not evaluated.	3 items from RMBPC Institutionalization at 6-mo. follow-up	---	FIM; 12-item QOL-AD; 16-item Agitated Behavior in Dementia Scale; Activity Engagement
CR results	CR of groups who received training (Tx 1 & 2 combined) had significantly delayed institutionalization compared to respite control. Survival analysis over 8 years indicates training resulted in CR remaining in home longer.	Not evaluated.	Significantly greater improvements among Hispanic/Latino and White/Cauc participants for CR problem behaviors, but not for Black/AA. Clinically significant improvements in problem behavior score for Latino/Hispanic. No differences in institutionalization at follow-up.	---	Adjusted mean difference (95%CI) at 4 months: Improvements in functional dependence: 0.24 (0.03-0.44); Improved engagement: 0.12 (0.07-0.22).

Study	Brodaty, et al. 1997[6]	Drummond, et al. 1991[9]	Belle, et al. 2006[10] REACH II	Holland, et al. 2009[11]	Gitlin, et al. 2010[12]
Comments	Residential program serving 4 CR-CG dyads at a time in small groups. Setting could be hotel or other grouping.	Economic analysis determined that the annual incremental cost of providing the support program was $2,204 (Canadian dollars) per caregiver, and that the improvement in CG QoL (as measured by the CQLI) was 0.11 over the 6-month intervention period. The implied incremental cost per QALY gained is therefore $2,204/0.11 or $20,036.	Stratified randomized assignment by site, ethnicity, and dyadic relationship. Follow-up limited to 6 mos., no 12 mo. data. According to authors: treatment is feasible in community settings delivered by BA in psychology, social work, nursing, OT or related.	Noncompleters similar to completers on care demographics. Universal, rather than targeted interventions, likely to show smaller effect sizes.	A high prevalence (close to 40%) was found of undiagnosed, treatable medical conditions among intervention CRs.

Abbreviations: AA = African American; ADL = activities of daily living; CES-D = Center for Epidemiologic Studies Depression Scale; CG = caregiver; CQLI = Caregiver Quality of Life Instrument; CR = care recipient; GQ-SR = good-quality systematic review; IADL = Instrumental Activities of Daily Living scale; ITT = intention-to-treat; PCI = patient care index; QALY = quality of adjusted life years; STAI = State Trait Anxiety Disorder; Tx 1 = treatment 1; Tx 2 = treatment 2.

EXERCISE TRAINING

Summary impact of exercise training interventions: There is insufficient evidence evaluating the impact of exercise for the CG on CG burden. More studies are needed.

One study, cited by two reviews, evaluated exercise training among 100 sedentary female CGs of a relative with dementia.[13] In this study, 51 CGs participated in a home-based exercise training program with 15 supportive telephone contacts, while 49 CGs received an attention-control condition in which CGs received supportive phone calls with nutrition guidance. The exercise training program successfully cultivated adherence to regular exercise participation, with a goal of four 30+ minute sessions per week, but demonstrated no effect on CG depression, stress, anxiety, or burden, compared with the controls. Both exercise and control groups demonstrated decreased depression, stress, and burden, but there were no significant differences between groups. The study authors noted that CGs who were more depressed at baseline demonstrated poorer adherence to the exercise regimen.[13]

CASE MANAGEMENT

Summary impact of case management interventions: Two RCTs published in 2006,[14, 15] which featured individualized assessment and care plans, report promising improvements in CG depression, stress, and confidence in caregiving, and reductions in CR problem behaviors. Prior to these studies there was little evidence to support that intensive nursing case management has a sustained impact on CG mood or strain. There may be some transience in the timing of beneficial effects, which were evident at some follow-up evaluations and not at others. There is insufficient evidence to support that case management interventions have an impact on rates of CR institutionalization.

Five studies investigated the impact of intensive nurse care case management on CG and CR outcomes, with mixed conclusions (Table 2). Three studies focused on institutionalization outcomes. Eloniemi-Sulkava and colleagues reported lower rates of institutionalization for the first months of the two year program among 53 individuals with dementia whose CGs received telephone and in-home support and psychoeducation, compared to usual care (N=47).[16] However, by the end of the two years there were no differences in rates of institutionalization between the intervention and control groups. The authors concluded that severely demented individuals on the verge of institutionalization would most benefit from this kind of program by delaying nursing home placement. Another study reported no evidence that nursing case management delayed institutionalization of the CR when compared to usual care.[17] An additional study apparently linked to the Miller, et al., database[18] reported there was no reduction in CG strain, burden, or depression resulting from nursing case management intervention that included respite care, home care, and consultation, but did find that the intervention group was more likely to use community services than the control group.

A fourth study provided collaborative care management for 84 CG-CR dyads with CG training in problem solving, behavior management, communication skills, and coping, as well as provision of advice, exercise guidelines, information on dementia, and invitation to voluntary support group sessions, compared to augmented usual care for 69 dyads, where primary care providers were permitted to refer for any treatments or services deemed appropriate.[14] Improvements related to intervention were intermittent but measurable; the authors reported significant intervention group improvements in CG stress as measured by the Neuropsychiatric Inventory for CGs, at 12 months follow-up but not 18 months. CGs under case management also endorsed improved mood on at 18 months compared to usual care control (but not at 6 or 12 months). CRs who participated in the intervention were rated with fewer total behavioral symptoms of dementia at the end of the study, but there was no impact on CR mood, cognition, or ability to complete ADL. The intervention did not influence likelihood of nursing home placement by the end of the study.

A fifth study included 408 CG-CR dyads, and demonstrated beneficial effects of individualized care management that provided teaching problem-solving skills, initiating care plan actions and generating a problem list for clinical care based on in-home structured assessment, compared to usual care.[15] Intervention CGs endorsed higher confidence in caregiving at 12 and 18 months, while mastery of caregiving skills and social support were rated as significantly improved over control at 18 months follow-up. CG health-related quality of life did not change as a result of the intervention. For CRs in the intervention group, there was nearly double the adherence to dementia treatment guidelines adopted *a priori* in the study protocol, and while health-related quality of life dropped for both groups, there was significantly less decline for the intervention participants. CGs also rated higher quality of health care for their CRs in the intervention group.

Limitations of the literature: The reduction in institutionalization in a population of community-dwelling elders in Finland[16] may not readily generalize to US or Veteran populations.

Table 2. RCTs of case management for caregivers of individuals with dementia

Study	Eloniemi-Sulkava, et al. 2001[16]	Miller, et al. 1999[17] MADDE study	Newcomer, et al. 1999[18]	Callahan, et al. 2006[14]	Vickrey, et al. 2006[15]
Population (N)	Community-living individuals with dementia and their unpaid family CGs. (N=100 dyads)	Community-dwelling CG-care recipient (CR) dyads where CR had dementia and CG was unpaid. (N=8095)	As in Miller, 1999.	Older adults with AD and their CGs. (N=153)	Informal CG-CR dyads from 18 primary care clinics. (N=408)
Intervention (N)	2-year nurse case management with support, education and cognitive training through telephone and in-home visits facilitated physician referrals, and 24-hour phone availability. (N=53)	Intensive case management, consultation, phone and in-home visits. Program also included respite care, home care, CR occupational therapy, CR nursing care, and case management. (N=4151)	As in Miller, 1999.	Collaborative care management including problem solving, behavior management training, communication skills training, coping skills training, advice, exercise guidelines, information on dementia, and invitation to voluntary support group sessions (attended at least once by 56%). (N=84)	Individualized care manager-led disease management intervention (teaching problem-solving skills, initiating care plan actions and generating a problem list for clinical care) following structured home assessment. Ongoing telephone follow-up with reassessment every 6 mos. (N=238)
Control (N)	Usual care. (N=47)	Usual care. (N=3944)	As in Miller, 1999.	Augmented usual care following any evaluation or treatment deemed appropriate by primary care provider. (N=69)	Usual care. (N=170)
CG outcome measures	Not evaluated.	Not evaluated. Zarit Burden Scale, Geriatric Depression Scale, and Zarit Stress Scale were measured as baseline covariates only.	Zarit Burden Scale Geriatric Depression Scale	NPI CG portion PHQ-9	CG knowledge of dementia (5 items) CG health
CG results	Not evaluated.	Not evaluated.	CM did not reduce strain or depression for CG.	Significant Intervention group improvements in CG stress at 12 mos. but not 18 mos. on NPI. Improved mood on PHQ9 at 18 months compared to usual care control (but not at 6 or 12 mos.).	Higher confidence in caregiving at 12 and 18 mos. Higher mastery of caregiving skills rated at 18 mos. Higher social support for Intervention group at 18 mos. Health related quality of life equivalent across groups.
CR outcome measures	Rate of institutionalization.	Rate of institutionalization.	Not evaluated.	NPI ADLs Health Care resource use CSDD Telephone Interview for Cognitive Status Medication List	Adherence to 23 guideline recommendations. Use of community resources. CR health CR quality of care

Study	Elomiemi-Sulkava, et al. 2001[16]	Miller, et al. 1999[17] MADDE study	Newcomer, et al. 1999[18]	Callahan, et al. 2006[14]	Vickrey, et al. 2006[15]
CR results	In early months of study, rate of CR institutionalization was lower in the intervention group. This effect was erased by the 24-month follow-up.	No significant differences in rate of institutionalization overall. Treatment was associated with increased rate of institutionalization (hazard rate 1.21, p=0.043) at 1 of 8 study sites.	Not evaluated.	Significant improvements in total NPI (fewer behavioral symptoms), No impact on CR depression, cognition, or function (ADLs). No influence of intervention on NH placement.	Intervention group had nearly doubled adherence to guidelines. Smaller decline in health-related quality of life for Intervention participants. CR Health care quality rated higher by CGs at 12 and 18 mos.
Comments	Population is Finnish, age 65+, living at home.	Study authors suggest that case managers at one site may have had a "stronger propensity to recommend nursing home placement than in the other sites," but reasons for why practices would differ were unclear.	Use of community services increased 50% with case management, compared to 40% increase in control participants.	---	Social workers were usually the care managers, feasibility enhanced by linking dyads to existing community resources rather than duplicating across systems.

Abbreviations: AA = African American; ADL = activities of daily living; CES-D = Center for Epidemiologic Studies Depression Scale; CG = caregiver; CQLI = Caregiver Quality of Life Instrument; CR = care recipient; GQ-SR = good-quality systematic review; IADL = Instrumental Activities of Daily Living scale; ITT = intention-to-treat; PCI = patient care index; QALY = quality of adjusted life years; STAI = State Trait Anxiety Disorder; Tx 1 = treatment 1; Tx 2 = treatment 2.

BEHAVIOR MANAGEMENT TRAINING (BMT)

Summary impact of behavior management training interventions: A limited body of evidence suggests that BMT may improve CG depression, although this finding was not consistent. Studies where BMT was augmented by CR exercise or CG self-care instruction seemed to result in broader outcome effects, improving CR physical mobility and CG coping skills.

Studies represented in this section specified the use of BMT, which involves identification of probable triggers and consequences of CR behavior disturbance and devising strategies to reduce the frequency of problem behaviors in the CR. Two of four studies provided BMT training to CGs with mixed results (Table 3). One study (N=95) comparing routine medical care with eight weekly in-home BMT sessions/four monthly telephone follow-up calls demonstrated improvements in CG subjective reports of depression and burden, as well as lowered reactivity to CR behavior disturbance and improved CR quality of life. This study also demonstrated that BMT is feasible in the primary care setting.[19] Another study (N=62) comparing four group trainings in behavioral interventions over eight weeks to an equivalent number of group sessions providing care-related discussions and advice found no treatment effects between groups, but reported significant pre to post improvement in CR aggression scores within the treatment group.[20]

A third study (N=153) offered a combined program of exercise for the person with dementia while supplying BMT for the CG, and reported improved physical health, increased activity, and decreased depression for the CR, as well as a trend toward lower institutionalization rates, compared to usual-care controls.[21] No outcomes were measured or reported for the CGs in this study. This combined approach may yield positive outcomes for both members of the dyad. However, it is not possible to separately evaluate the efficacy of the treatment components, as the intervention group combined both BMT for the CG and exercise for the CR.[21]

One study educated 37 CGs on behavior management techniques through instructive pamphlets and compared that basic intervention with an enhanced intervention (N=39) that added pamphlets on CG self-care.[22] CGs in the enhanced care group demonstrated significantly higher ratings of general well-being after two years of intervention, but found no effects on CG mood.

In addition to the RCTs identified from previous systematic reviews, we included three good quality studies[23-25] found in the AoA compendium.[2] One study demonstrated the applicability of BMT interventions with Chinese-American CGs (N=55), resulting in less bother and lower depression for the treatment group but no difference in overall reported stress.[23] Another study (N = 80) reported significantly lower CG distress about CR neuropsychiatric symptoms, but no change in burden for either treatment or control group.[24] The third study of 143 CGs reported that the CG treatment group had reduced emotional distress over CR agitated behaviors over time (compared to baseline), but there was no overall group effect for treatment on distress scores.[25] The findings of these three studies are relatively consistent with those reported in previous studies.

Limitations of the literature: There was an overall lack of methodologic rigor, and only one study stipulated statistical considerations such as the power to detect a treatment difference or intention-to-treat analysis.[19, 21] Heterogeneity in the interventions delivered makes it difficult to combine findings across studies.

Table 3. RCTs of behavioral management training for caregivers of individuals with dementia

Study	Teri, et al. 2005[19]	Teri, et al. 2003[21]	Gormley, et al. 2001[20]	Burns, et al. 2003[22]
Population (N)	95 family CGs of patients with AD.	153 CG living with CR who met NINCDS/ADRDA criteria for AD, randomly assigned to intervention or control.	62 individuals with dementia living with their CG.	167 dyads of indiv2duals with dementia and their CG randomized to Behavior Care or Enhanced Care. After 24 months, 76 pairs remained active, 30 bereaved, 14 placed in long-term care, and 47 lost to follow-up.
Specific intervention (N)	In-home BMT training for CG in 8 weekly sessions, and 4 monthly follow-up calls.	Combined exercise and CG in-home training in behavior management program "Reducing Disability in Alzheimer Disease" for 3 months. (N=76)	4 group sessions over 8 weeks teaching behavioral interventions to CG including acting at level of precipitating and maintaining factors, using appropriate communication, accepting false statements by CR (not arguing), and using distraction techniques. Additional problem-solving for unsuccessful interventions. (N=34)	Enhanced Care provided same Behavior Care as control but with 12 additional pamphlets focused on improving well-being of CG, presented during primary care visits by masters-level health educator. Sessions no longer than 60 minutes, with 10-minute phone contacts between sessions. (N =39)
Control (N)	Routine medical care with no specific BMT.	Routine medical care. (N=77)	Equivalent number of group sessions consisting of care-related discussions and advice about available services. (N=28)	Behavior Care provided 25 pamphlets focused on improving BMT repertoire of CG, presented during primary care visits by masters-level health educator. Sessions no longer than 30 minutes, with 10-minute phone contacts between sessions. (N=37)
CG outcome measures	CES-D HDRS Caregiver Sleep Questionnaire Perceived Stress Scale Screen for Caregiver Burden SSCQ	Not evaluated.	ZBI	General Well-Being Scale CES-D RMBPC
CG results	Significantly greater improvements in depression, burden, and reactivity to CR behavior problems at 2 and 6-month post-tests for intervention group; improvements in sleep quality at 6-month follow-up for intervention group.	Not evaluated.	No significant differences between groups in ZBI score post-intervention.	Enhanced Care group showed less bother (RMBPC) at baseline. Lower income and less education at baseline for Enhanced Care participants were controlled in subsequent analyses. General well-being improved significantly for Enhanced Care group over 2 years relative to Behavior Care group; but both groups improved. No significant group benefits over time for depression or risk of depression, though trends suggest possible benefit of Enhanced Care for mood over time.

Interventions for Non-professional Caregivers of Individuals with Dementia

Study	Teri, et al. 2005[19]	Teri, et al. 2003[21]	Gormley, et al. 2001[20]	Burns, et al. 2003[22]
CR outcome measures	NPI RMBPC QOL-AD	Physical mobility, depression, and institutionalization (MMSE, SF-36, SIP mobility, HDRS, CSDD, RMB-PC, adverse symptom checklist)	BEHAVE-AD RAGE MMSE BDRS	Katz ADL scale, Lawton and Brody IADL scale, and MMSE were collected as part of the larger REACH battery.
CR results	Improved CG ratings of CR quality of life for intervention group at 2-month follow-up; similar trend at 6 months that was significant when controlled for differences in ethnicity.	Compared to routine care, significantly improved scores for physical functioning in intervention group at 3-month and 2-year follow-up, and significantly improved depression (based on direct rater observation and CG interviews) at 3 months. Less institutionalization due to behavior disturbance at 2 years for intervention group, statistically not significant. Higher baseline depression scores predicted significant improvement of intervention over control group at 3-month and 2-year follow-ups.	Baseline RAGE scores were modestly higher in the intervention group with no significant group differences in post treatment aggression scores. Within the intervention group, there was significant reduction in RAGE score from pre to post, but not within the control group. No significant changes in psychotropic prescribing for either group.	Not reported.
Comments	Copy of treatment manual available from Dr. Teri. Somewhat resource-intensive training and supervision of behavior consultants, but could be implemented by VA staff psychologists and social workers.	Results can only be generalized as combined effect, as relative contributions of BMT and exercise were not evaluated.	Difference reported within group, but this analysis loses benefit of randomization. Comparison between randomized groups yielded no significant differences. Evidence from this study is not strong.	No ITT analysis, but shorter length of time performing CG duties was only difference between completers and noncompleters. Blinding not part of protocol.

Abbreviations: AD = Alzheimer's disease; ADL = activities of daily living; ADRDA = Alzheimer Disease and Related Disorders Association; BDRS = Blessed Dementia Rating Scale; BEHAVE-AD = Behavioral Pathology in Alzheimer's Disease rating scale; CES-D = Center for Epidemiologic Studies Depression Scale; CG = caregiver; CR = care recipient; CSDD = Cornell Scale for Depression and Dementia; GQ-SR = good-quality systematic review; HDRS = Hamilton Depression Rating Scale; IADL = Instrumental Activities of Daily Living scale; ITT = intention-to-treat; MMSE = Mini Mental State Exam; NINCDS = National Institute of Neurological and Communicative Diseases and Stroke; NPI = Neuropsychiatric Inventory; QOL-AD = Quality of Life in Alzheimer's Disease; RMBPC = Revised Memory and Behavior Problem Checklist; SF-36 = Short-form health survey; SIP = Sickness Impact Profile; SSCQ = Short Sense of Competence Questionnaire; ZBI = Zarit Burden Interview.

INDIVIDUAL SKILLS TRAINING

Summary impact of individual skills training interventions: Most studies found no impact on CG's sense of burden, anxiety, or quality of life, though two of six studies demonstrated that individual skills training for the CG ameliorates depression in CGs. CRs may benefit with slower declines in self-care when skills training includes a component targeting their ADL, and improved mood when pleasant events are scheduled, but these findings were not replicated in other studies. Two of six studies reported that disruptive behavior may be reduced when CGs receive structured training in identifying triggers of disruptive behavior and modifying the environment to reduce stress. There is no consistent evidence documenting impact of skills training programs on delaying or preventing institutionalization of the CR.

Six studies where CGs were taught new skills during individual interactions between the CG and study staff are described here. These interventions typically focused on combinations of: increasing the CG's repertoire of problem solving strategies, modifying the environment to decrease hazard and reduce triggers of problem behaviors, and/or increasing CG's sense of support and self-efficacy (Table 4a).

The studies on individual skills training allowed for examination of specific CG outcomes across studies, such as depression, mood, and other CG problems. A summary of the findings on specific CG outcomes are presented below.

CG depression outcomes. Two studies found significant reduction in CGs' reported depressive symptoms. Buckwalter, et al. compared controls receiving two informational home visits and reading material about dementia to an intervention of in-home training to reduce environmental stressors followed by phone consultation.[26] The intervention resulted in reduced depressive symptoms at six months but *not* at 12 month follow-up. The second study examined individualized phone consultation focused on increasing self-efficacy compared with usual care.[27] Self-reported CG depression scores improved with intervention, which also significantly increased CG reports of perceived self-efficacy. This study also reported higher CG satisfaction with care when telephone consults targeted self-efficacy.

Outcomes for other CG problems. Reduction in negative CG responses such as anger[26] or upset/aversive response to problem behaviors[28, 29] was reported for three programs that targeted environmental stressors through structured home visits.

Mood and problem behavior outcomes for CR. Some CG skills training studies reported significant improvements for CRs. One study focused on increasing the number of pleasant events scheduled for CRs, combined with teaching problem solving strategies to CGs, resulting in significant improvement in CG *and* CR ratings of the CR's mood/depression.[30] One study reported less decline in self-care for the CR under a protocol that provided occupational therapist home visits teaching problem solving to the CG for behavioral triggers, combined with training for the CR in performingADL.[29] Two studies[28, 29] reported significant reductions in CR behavior disturbance, but in one study this finding only held for dyads with non-spouse CGs.[28] One study reported a significantly larger proportion of CRs remained at home at 12 month follow-up when their CGs received nurse's individual supportive counseling and strategies for behavior management, compared to controls who received phone contacts at comparably scheduled time points.[31] However, there were no differences between groups in numbers of CRs *institutionalized* at this same follow-up, possibly indicating differences between groups at baseline, or other factors such as CR mortality, impacting on proportions remaining at home.

Limitations of the literature: There is some likely overlap between training offered in these studies and the clearly defined behavior management training techniques outlined in another section. For the most part, these good quality studies were well-controlled and characterized by intention to treat analysis when possible. There were high loss-to-follow-up rates in two studies, though they were not different in intervention and controls. However, unequal sample sizes, varying measures across studies, and differing recruitment strategies – some drawing from populations seeking help for dementia-related problems and others drawing from clinic populations – were common limitations.

Interventions for Non-professional Caregivers of Individuals with Dementia

Table 4a. RCTs of individual skills training for caregivers of individuals with dementia

Study	Teri, et al. 1997[30]	Gitlin, et al. 2001[29]	Buckwalter, et al. 1999[26]	Gerdner, et al. 2002[28]	Wright, et al. 2001[31]	Bass, et al. 2003[27]
Population (N)	Individuals with dementia and their co-resident community CGs. 88 pairs began the study, 72 (82%) completed.	Dementia patients with ADL dependence in 2 areas, difficult behavior and their family CGs. (N=171)	Informal CGs of community-dwelling individual with dementia or memory impairment. (N=245 completed study, missing data for 5, attrition of 28%)	Home CGs of individuals with Alzheimer's disease. (N=241 yielding 237 complete records)	Family CGs of individuals with dementia previously treated for agitation. (N=93)	Primary family CGs of Kaiser patients who had dementia or memory loss coded in medical record. (N=182 completed first interview, 157 of those also completed 12-month follow-up interview)
Intervention (N)	Two active behavioral treatments involving CG skills training: increasing patient pleasant events (nine 60-minute weekly sessions, N = 23) and CG problem solving strategies without pleasant events focus. (N = 19)	Five home visits by occupational therapists providing CG skills training (environmental modifications, avoiding overstimulation, etc.) and CR ADL training. (N=93)	Progressively Lowered Stress Threshold model of care, individually tailored to problems in the home. Provided 3-4 hours of in-home training and bi-weekly follow-up phone calls for 6 months. (N=132)	Same as control plus individualized care plan presented at 2 in-home visits, 2 weeks apart, building structured routine for CR and modification of environmental challenges (reduce water temperature to prevent scalding, remove mirrors to reduce visual confusion). (N=132)	Individual supportive counseling and strategies for behavior management by nurse after baseline assessment during inpatient admission for 3 home visits (2, 6, and 12 weeks), then 2 phone follow-ups at 6 and 12 months post discharge. (N=68)	Telephone care consultation intervention by Alzheimer's Association staff. Individual care plan outlines tasks and timelines. Biweekly follow-ups decreasing to 1 and 3-month intervals, adjusted as needed. (60% of sample; N not reported.)
Control (N)	Equal duration typical care, unstructured information, and support for solving patient problems (N = 10), and wait-list control receiving no contact during the 9 week period. (N = 20)	No intervention, provided education materials and a safety booklet at the end of the study. (N=78)	Two in-home visits providing general information about dementia, referral to community-based services and groups, and reading material about dementia. Similar phone follow-up. (N=108)	Receipt of routine information and referrals for community-based services, case management and support groups, provided at 2 one-hour visits, 2 weeks apart. (N=105)	Contact by phone for data collection only, same time points as intervention group. (N=25)	Usual managed care services. (40% of sample; N not reported.)
CG outcome measures	SADS; Hamilton DRS was derived from SADS score; ZBI	Measured CG ratings of self efficacy and upset in managing dementia behavior.	POMS; GDRS	Caregiver response to behavior problems.	Caregiver Hassle Scale; CES-D; MAI	T1 and T2 interviews: A 2-item index of satisfaction with the types of Kaiser services; an 8-item index of satisfaction with the quality of Kaiser services; a 5-item index of satisfaction with information received about the illness; CG depression measure similar to CES-D.

Study	Teri et al. 1997[30]	Gitlin, et al. 2001[29]	Buckwalter, et al. 1999[26]	Gerdner, et al. 2002[28]	Wright, et al. 2001[31]	Bass, et al. 2003[27]
CG results	CG depression decreased significantly in both treatment groups compared with control conditions. CG results were similar between the 2 active treatment conditions (pleasant events vs. problem solving).	Reduced upset. Women reported increased self-efficacy in managing behaviors, and women and minors reported enhanced self-efficacy in managing functional dependency.	Significantly less depression in intervention group at 6 months, but not at 12-month follow-up. Anger-hostility, fatigue-inertia, confusion-bewilderment, all significantly lower for intervention group than control at both 6 and 12-month follow-up.	CGs in intervention group had less aversive response to memory/behavioral problems than control participants. Spouses' response to activities of daily living problems improved with intervention condition.	No effect was demonstrated.	Significantly less CG depression (11 items from CES-D) in intervention vs. control. CGs in intervention group whose CR had not received specific dementia diagnosis rated higher levels of satisfaction with service quality, types of services, and information about the illness.
CR outcome measures	HDRS CSDD BDI MMSE DRS RIL	MBPC FIM	Not evaluated.	MBPC	BDRS CMAI	During a 1-year period: number of hospital admissions, emergency department visits, physician visits, and Kaiser case management visits
CR results	CR depression significantly responded to the 2 treatment conditions compared with the control conditions. CR results were similar between the two active treatment conditions (pleasant events vs. problem solving).	Fewer declines in IADLs and self-care, and fewer behavior problems in intervention group compared with controls at 3-month post-test.	Not evaluated.	Effect of intervention on frequency of behavioral disturbance significant for non-spouse (younger) CGs only.	More CRs remained at home at 12-month follow-up in the intervention group (61% vs. 56% of control CRs), but proportionally fewer deaths in the treatment group (11% vs. 22%) may have contributed to this effect. The proportion institutionalized did not significantly differ between groups (28% Tx vs. 22% controls).	Less use of Kaiser case management and direct care community services with intervention. Less use of non-Alzheimer's Association information and support services for patients with more severe memory problems with intervention. No differences in use of emergency department, hospital admissions and physician visits.

26

Study	Teri, et al. 1997[30]	Gitlin, et al. 2001[29]	Buckwalter, et al. 1999[26]	Gerdner, et al. 2002[28]	Wright, et al. 2001[31]	Bass, et al. 2003[27]
Comments	No significant differences between baseline measures of completers and noncompleters.	ITT analysis; baseline recorded blind before group assignment.	CGs who were more depressed were more likely to drop out between 6 and 12 months, and institutionalization of their CR more likely. High attrition (28%) but no differential loss to follow-up.	Very high attrition (54%); similar in treatment groups and across research sites. The beneficial effect of the intervention on negative CG reactions was greater among spousal compared with non-spousal CGs.	Large difference in group sizes may have contributed to Type II error.	Physicians and managed care providers blinded to group assignment. Population drawn from primary care and not limited to those seeking help with dementia-related problems.

Abbreviations: ADL = activities of daily living; BDI = Beck Depression Inventory; BDRS = Blessed Dementia Rating Scale; CES-D = Center for Epidemiologic Studies Depression Scale; CG = caregiver; CMAI = Cohen-Mansfield Agitation Inventory; CR = care recipient; CSDD = Cornell Scale for Depression and Dementia; DRS = Dementia Rating Scale; FIM = Functional Independence Measure; GDRS = Geriatric Depression Rating Scale; HDRS = Hamilton Depression Rating Scale; IADL = Instrumental Activities of Daily Living scale; MAI = Multilevel Assessment Inventory; MBPC = Memory and Behavior Problems Checklist; MMSE = Mini Mental State Exam; POMS = Profile of Moods States; RIL = Record of Independent Living; SADS = Social Avoidance and Distress Scale; SR = systematic review; T1 = timepoint 1; T2 = timepoint 2; ZBI = Zarit Burden Interview.

Columns separated by a dashed line indicate that the two publications appear to be related and may be based on the same study

GROUP SKILLS TRAINING, AND
COMBINED INDIVIDUAL/GROUP SKILLS TRAINING

Summary impact of group skills training interventions: There is evidence that CG depression may improve with interventions that are individualized by in-home assessment and targeted to specific needs of the patient-CG dyad. Ancillary improvements in positive interactions and nurturing, reducing aversive and hostile CG responses to problem behaviors, reducing CG burden, and increasing CG self-efficacy are supported by single studies in the skills training domain.

Eight studies included in this grouping reported specific attempts to teach CGs new skills in group,[32-36] combined individual/group settings,[37, 38] or group sessions combined with transportable training media.[39] Skills training included management of CR behavior problems, CG stress, or identifying environmental problems such as poor lighting that might contribute to CR strain or injury, and most interventions also provided psychoeducation about dementia. Two studies were conducted in the same sample.[34, 35]

The studies on group skills training and combined individual/group skills training allowed for examination of specific CG outcomes across studies, such as depression, mood, and other CG problems (Tables 4b and 4c). A summary of the findings on specific CG outcomes are presented below.

CG depression. CGs who received the intervention rated improved mood over control conditions in three of the six studies. A study of the Minnesota Family Workshop (MFW) program provided 14 hours of group skills training sessions to 75 CGs to increase coping and stress management skills; educate about dementia; and develop care strategies, compared to 45 participants in a wait-list control condition.[34] This intervention resulted in significant improvement in self-ratings of CG burden, sense of nurturing, and aversive response to CR behavior. A subsequent study (N−215) by the same investigators assessed the long-term effects of a MFW-based program on CG distress, and found treatment benefits in CG attitude and distress at six months, but these effects were no longer significant at one year.[36] In another study, parallel intervention groups (one focused on anger management cognitive-behavioral intervention and one focused on depression cognitive-behavioral intervention) were compared to wait-list control with resulting significant reductions in depression and anger/hostility for both interventions compared to control.[32] A third study investigated the impact of two distinct training groups, the first trained CGs to use behavior management techniques to reduce CR aversive behaviors, the alternate group taught CGs to change their own coping behaviors.[37] Both interventions combined individualized in-home assessment and trainings with a three-hour group workshop to teach CG skills identified by the assessment. Both intervention groups were compared to a control group that received similarly scheduled workshops and in home visits with supportive empathy, but the didactics were general (e.g., information about stages of dementia) rather than individualized. The "self-change" group reflected significant improvements in CG depression at post-test, three month, and six month follow-up, while the "patient change" intervention resulted in significant CG depression reductions at post-test and six-month follow-up. Both intervention groups also rated improvements over control group participants in patient problem behaviors at posttest and six months, with the "patient change" group additionally documenting reduced problem behaviors at three months.

CG satisfaction with CR interactions. One study provided group workshops training CGs to stimulate the minds of their CR, and compared outcomes to a placebo group organized around a passive activity (e.g., watching television) and a control group that received assessment contacts only. On follow-up measures, CGs in the intervention group reported significantly higher satisfaction with interactions with the CR, though there were no significant effects for improved mood, burden, or quality of life.[33]

Other CG outcomes. One study combined a group workshop teaching stress management skills, with eight in-home behavior-management sessions, and compared this to minimal support control in which CGs were provided brief, structured telephone support calls with a target time of 15 minutes per call.[38] Both intervention and control groups improved significantly over baseline measures, reporting less bother, increased satisfaction, and fewer problem behaviors at six-month post-test. An analysis by race determined that the skills-training intervention was more effective for reducing bother among African American CGs, whereas the minimal support control condition was more effective for White CGs. African American CGs were significantly less receptive to the minimal support phone contacts, with calls lasting an average of two fewer minutes in duration compared with calls to White CGs. The desire to institutionalize differed by race independently of intervention group: desire to institutionalize increased among White CGs, while scores for African American CGs on this measure remained stable.[38]

We examined an additional group skills training intervention suggested by a technical reviewer. The Savvy Caregiver Program is a transportable, packaged program for CGs of adults with dementia modeled on the MFW program.[40] The package includes a trainer's manual, a CG's manual, and a CD-ROM or videotape meant to complement the CG manual. The program could be offered in the community by governmental, educational, medical, or social service provider organizations, and involves six two-hour group sessions led by a trainer with an educational or clinical background. A randomized trial of the Savvy Caregiver program included 52 CGs in three states, and assessed CG psychosocial outcomes after six months.[39] The study reported significantly improved scores on measures of confidence and distress among CGs in the intervention group compared with wait-list controls. The attrition rate was high (nearly 50%), however, and the study authors cited logistic difficulties in retaining participation and collecting data. Although the generalizability of this study is consequently limited, the promising findings warrant more rigorous investigation of this packaged program on a larger scale.

Limitations of the literature: The studies reviewed here represent skills-focused training in groups or combined with individual training, but there is likely to be considerable variability in methods and deployment of the groups. The skill level of the trainer, the setting, frequency and duration of contacts, the validity of the training material and relevance to the outcome variables of interest, and method of recruitment are likely to contribute to unmeasured variance and differences in outcomes across studies. Intervention and control group sizes tended to be small and loss-to-follow-up high, a situation common to studies with frail and/or distressed populations. Studies tended to differ on policy for inclusion/exclusion of data from follow-up analyses if the CR had died during the study; the degree to which this could confound measures such as burden and depression is suspect but unknown.

Table 4b. RCTs of group skills training for caregivers of individuals with dementia

Study	Corbeil, et al. 1999[33]	Hepburn, et al. 2007 (The Savvy Caregiver Program)[39]	Hepburn, et al. 2006 (Partners in Caregiving)[36]	Hepburn, et al. 2001 (The Minnesota Family Workshop)[34]	Ostwald, et al. 1999[35]	Coon, et al. 2003[32]
Population (N)	Coresident CGs of patients with probable or possible Alzheimer's dementia with mild-moderate functional impairments. (N=87)	Family CGs of older adults with dementia recruited by agencies in 3 states.(N=30) There were 9 Savvy CG programs ranging from 3 to 10 CGs.	215 CGs giving care to a community-dwelling relative with dementia, who were expecting their CR to remain in the community for the 1 year study duration.	Primary CGs of community-dwelling individuals with dementia. (N=117)	Primary CGs of community-dwelling individuals with dementia who had displayed behavior problems. (N=117 of whom 94 dyads completed the program.)	Female CGs of community-dwelling individuals with physician-confirmed dementia (primarily Alzheimer's and stroke). (N=169)
Intervention (N)	Active cognitive stimulation: 1-hour group sessions for 12 weeks, 6 days/week, offering training in activities to stimulate the minds of the CR. (N=28)	A 6-session, packaged program derived from the Minnesota Family Workshop that includes a trainer's manual, CG manual, and CD-ROM or videotape. The packaged program can be offered by a variety of organizations or groups, with leadership typically provided by persons with an educational or clinical background.	Tx 1: Day-to-day caregiving (N=79) Tx 2: Decision-making (N=72) Each group met for 2 hours per week over 6 consecutive weeks. Curricula focused on developing a more clinical perspective on caregiving. Content and results were similar between Tx groups, and data were combined in the analysis.	Seven weekly training groups to improve coping and stress management; provision of information about dementia, develop strategies for care. Follow-up measures at 3 months after last training. (N=72)	Seven weekly training groups to improve coping and stress management; provision of information about dementia, develop strategies for care. Follow-up measures at 3 months after last training. (N=60)	Two intervention groups: 1) Anger management cognitive-based training (N=41) 2) Depression management cognitive behavioral training (N=45) - 8, 2-hour weekly group sessions, followed by 2 monthly booster sessions.
Control (N)	Passive stimulation: placebo intervention that included only passive activities (e.g. television) but had the same exposure to the researchers and followed the same time frames (television). (N=28) Wait-list control: interactions limited to 3 assessment contacts only; intervention was offered after 9-month study time frame. (N=31)	Wait-listed, no-attention control group (N=22), who were offered the training sessions after the 6-month intervention period.	Wait-list, no attention control group (N=64) with no contact with study staff except for data collection. Controls were enrolled in a PIC program after the completion of one-year data collection.	5-6 month wait-list control. (N=45) Control group CGs participated in the training intervention after data had been gathered from the treatment group CGs.	5-6 month wait-list control (N=34)	Wait-list control with initial assessment, 3-4 month follow-up assessment, and brief intermittent phone calls to maintain interest in study. Opportunity to participate in choice of intervention at end of 2nd assessment. (N=44)

Interventions for Non-professional Caregivers of Individuals with Dementia

Study	Corbeil, et al. 1999[33]	Hepburn, et al. 2007 (The Savvy Caregiver Program)[39]	Hepburn, et al. 2006 (Partners in Caregiving)[36]	Hepburn, et al. 2001 (The Minnesota Family Workshop)[34]	Ostwald, et al. 1999[35]	Coon, et al. 2003[32]
CG outcome measures	Ways of Coping Scale-Revised, Social Support Questionnaire of Schaefer, Zarit Marital Needs Satisfaction Scale	A composite distress score computed as a weighted composite of 12 scales that include CES-D, Zarit Burden Scale, Bradburn affect scale, REACH anxiety scale	CES-D, Zarit Burden Scale, STAI, BACS, Decisional Conflict Scale, Composite measure for distress	RMBPC, BACS, CES-D, Zarit Burden Scale	CES-D, Revised Caregiver Burden Scale, RMBPC	RSCSE, STAXI, MAACL, Ways of Coping Checklist-Revised, BDI
CG results	At 9-month follow-up, CG satisfaction remained positive in the intervention group, but became negative in both the wait-list control and passive (placebo) groups. This improvement was statistically significant.	Distress at 6 months did not change among control CGs but decreased significantly among CGs in the Tx group. Tx CGs also reported a significantly greater sense of mastery (confidence) at 6 months.	Distress level increased and attitude about caregiving worsened among control CGs but remained stable at 6 months among Tx CGs. These advantages were no longer significant at 12 months.	Within treatment group, significant pre-post increase in nurturing score (less subordination of self to CR) and decreased reaction to behavior disturbance of CR. Compared to control group, intervention CG demonstrated increased nurturing, decreased reaction to behavior, lower depression and burden.	Reduced negative reaction to disruptive behavior and reduced burden in intervention group.	Significant reductions in anger/hostility and depression, and increase in self-efficacy in both intervention groups relative to control participants.
CR outcome measures	Memory and Behavioral Problems Checklist: measured as stressors for analysis of CG outcomes; not evaluated as outcomes of the intervention	ADL/IADL and disruptive behaviors measured as covariates; not evaluated as outcomes of the intervention.	---	MMSE, Lawton ADL, and RMBPC were measured as covariates; not evaluated as outcomes of the intervention.	Cognitive Performance Test, MMSE, RMBPC	Not evaluated.
CR results	Not evaluated.	Not evaluated.	---	Not evaluated.	No reduction in disruptive behaviors.	Not evaluated.
Comments	Small group sizes.	High attrition: 102 CGs were recruited into the study and completed baseline questionnaires, but only 51% retention and follow-up was achieved.	The study authors combined established scales to develop a composite distress measure; study author comments that the measure needs further testing and development.	Small sample. Population accessed as result of request for help with problem.	Dropouts and completers comparable on baseline demographics except for patient age.	Small but significant effect sizes. Participants not recruited from distressed population. Participation limited to women.

Abbreviations: ADL = activities of daily living; BDI = Beck Depression Inventory; BDRS = Blessed Dementia Rating Scale; CES-D = Center for Epidemiologic Studies Depression Scale; CG = caregiver; CMAI = Cohen-Mansfield Agitation Inventory; CR = care recipient; CSDD = Cornell Scale for Depression and Dementia; DRS = Dementia Rating Scale; FIM = Functional Independence Measure; GDRS = Geriatric Depression Rating Scale; HDRS = Hamilton Depression Rating Scale; IADL = Instrumental Activities of Daily Living scale; MAI = Multilevel Assessment Inventory; MBPC = Memory and Behavior Problems Checklist; MMSE = Mini Mental State Exam; POMS = Profile of Moods States; RIL = Record of Independent Living; SADS = Social Avoidance and Distress Scale; SR = systematic review; T1 = timepoint 1; T2 = timepoint 2; ZBI = Zarit Burden Interview.

Columns separated by a dashed line indicate that the two publications appear to be related and may be based on the same study.

Table 4c. RCTs of combined individual skills training and group workshops for caregivers of individuals with dementia

Study	Bourgeois, et al. 2002[37]	Burgio, et al. 2003[38]
Population (N)	Patients meeting NINCDS-ADRDA criteria for probable AD who also had mild behavioral disturbance, and their primary (spouse spending at least 8 hours per day with CR) and secondary (identified by primary CG, spent minimum 4 hours per day with patient) CGs. (N=76 enrolled, 63 completed the intervention period)	White and African American CGs of individuals with dementia and at least 3 problem behaviors. (N=118)
Intervention (N)	Two distinct 12-week skills training groups: 1) train CG to change CR behavior (N = 22); and 2) train CG to change own coping behaviors (N = 21). Initial meetings individual at-home assessment for two 1-hour visits, then 3-hour workshop in group, then 9 in-home visits for skills training. Follow-up measures 3 and 6 months post intervention.	Stress management and BMT skills training through group workshop, then 8 in-home BMT and cognitive restructuring sessions.
Control (N)	Comparable attention at workshops and in-home visits, but no training except didactics on stages of adjustment to dementia (and Problem Behavior Tracking forms reviewed at home visits. Provided generalized rather than individual information and empathy). (N=20)	Minimal support control.
CG outcome measures	Caregiver Strain Scale Spielberger Anger Expression Scale Spielberger Anxiety Inventory Caregiver Self-Efficacy Assessment Perceived Stress Scale CES-D Caregiver Health Index Caregiver mood - single item on a scale (1-9)	PAC LSNI CES-D
CG results	Mood ratings improved relative to controls in "self-change" CG group at post-test and 3 and 6-month follow-ups. Mood improved for "patient change" CGs relative to controls at posttest and 6-month follow-up.	No changes in depression or anxiety over 6 months. Both groups improved, reporting less bother and increased satisfaction with leisure activities.
CR outcome measures	MMSE OARS BEHAVE-AD	RMBPC
CR results	Reduced mean frequency of problem behaviors in "change patient behavior" group compared to control at post-test and 3 and 6-month follow-up. Reduction in behavior problems for "self-change" CG group at post-test and 6-month follow-up.	Significantly fewer problem behaviors in the CR were noted by CGs in both treatment and control groups.
Comments	Research assistants blinded to group assignment administered measurements. Results indicate that dyads might benefit most from interventions specifically targeted to their needs (CG mood vs. care recipient behavior disturbance).	Staff not blinded to group assignment, but assessment and intervention always conducted by separate individuals. Six-month follow-up data include measures from CG whose CR had died – therefore, sample size changes on measures that were no longer appropriate. Different effects for African American versus White, and spouse vs. nonspouse CGs in secondary analyses.

Abbreviations: BEHAVE-AD = Behavioral Pathology in Alzheimer's Disease rating scale; BMT = Behavior Management Training; CES-D = Center for Epidemiologic Studies Depression Scale; CG = caregiver; CR = care recipient; GQ-SR = good-quality systematic review; LSNI = Lubben Social Network Index; MMSE = Mini Mental State Exam; NINCDS-ADRDA = National Institute of Neurological and Communicative Diseases and Stroke – Alzheimer Disease and Related Disorders Association; OARS = Older Americans Resource and Services Multidimensional Functional Assessment Questionnaire; PAC = Positive Aspects of Caregiving scale; RMBPC = Revised Memory and Behavior Problem Checklist.

INDIVIDUAL, GROUP, AND COMBINED INDIVIDUAL/GROUP SUPPORTIVE COUNSELING

Summary impact of individual, group, and combined individual/group supportive counseling interventions: Neither individual supportive counseling nor group supportive interventions on their own demonstrated clear superiority over control groups for CG depression. A combined individual/group approach resulted in delayed institutionalization for the CR and long-term improvements in mood and self-rated health for the CG, but this was a very resource-intensive intervention and replicability should be evaluated.[41-44] Ancillary improvements in affective regulation for coping and aversive reaction to CR behavior disturbance were supported in single studies. None of these interventions demonstrated group treatment effects for CG burden.

Studies were included in this group when supportive behaviors were an intentional focus of treatment. Six studies in this collection employed supportive interventions, including empathy, emotional support, and identifying sources of support in the environment.[41-43, 45-47]

One of the six studies reported on *individual* supportive counseling with cognitive-behavioral problem solving focus by a nurse care manager.[45] Two studies focused on CG *group* counseling protocols with: education about dementia, problem-solving, stress management, provision of emotional support, cognitive reappraisal;[46] and coping strategies, problem-solving, and identifying social supports.[47] These three studies are shown in Table 5a. There were no significant treatment effects on CG depression, burden, or anxiety for any of these three studies. However, Haley and colleagues reported that CGs trained in affective regulation for coping showed significant improvements in affective regulation,[46] and Hebert, et al. documented significantly less CG aversive reaction to CR behavior disturbance with coping/problem-solving supportive interventions.[47]

Three studies that combined individual counseling and support group sessions are shown in Table 5b. One study by Zarit, Anthony, & Boutselis (N=119) compared an intervention combining eight weeks of individual and family therapy, to eight weekly support group sessions, with both compared to wait list control (eight weeks, then enrollment into group).[48] All groups, including the control arm, responded with improved mood and burden; there were no group treatment effects.

In a series of reports, Mittelman and colleagues reported on a trial of the New York University Caregiver Intervention conducted between 1987 and 2006. The intervention involved four months of individual family counseling followed by weekly support groups offering psychoeducation on BMT, identifying social supports, and enhancing communication, compared to usual care at an Alzheimer's Disease Center.[41-43, 49] CGs in these studies responded to the intervention with significantly reduced depression, sustained as long as three years into follow-up.[42, 43] This approach combining individualized assessment with supportive group sessions also significantly reduced risk of institutionalization for the CR, with longer median length of stay in the home compared to usual care.[41, 49] The initial analyses included 206 CGs,[41, 43] and subsequent analyses of the continuing trial (N=406) reported long-term improvements for the CG in social support, stress appraisals, and self-rated health, as well as delayed nursing home placement for the CR.[42, 44, 49]

Limitations of the literature: There is definitional and functional overlap with case management, BMT, and skills-focused studies reported earlier; supportive counseling often included problem-solving and teaching of skills, and all interventions likely included some element of supportive empathy, even when that was not the targeted intervention. Some studies excluded CGs whose loved one was institutionalized or had died during the study from the final analysis, while others included some but not all CGs who no longer had a CR with dementia in the home at the time of final follow-up measurement. Recruitment strategies differed in that some studies sampled from CG populations that were seeking help for an identified behavior problem, while others drew from a more general Alzheimer's Association or dementia clinic population.

Table 5a. RCTs of individual counseling or group support for caregivers of individuals with dementia

Study	Roberts, et al. 1999[45]	Haley, Brown & Levine 1987[46]	Heber, et al. 2003[47]
Population (N)	CGs of cognitively-impaired home-dwelling individuals. (N=77)	Family CGs of community-dwelling individuals with dementia. (N=54)	Primary CGs of community dwelling individuals with dementia and one+ behavior problem; CGs report moderate to severe burden on scale. (N=118 in final analysis after death and institutionalization of 25 CR)
Intervention (N)	Individual counseling: Nurse provided up to 10 supportive, individualized problem-solving (cognitive behavioral) counseling sessions over 6 months. Measures at baseline, 6 and 12 months. (N=38)	Group 1: structured provision of information about dementia, emotional support, and problem solving. (N=21) Group 2: similar to Group 1 but added material on stress-management, relaxation, cognitive reappraisal. (N=22) Both groups: 7 weekly 1.5 hour sessions followed by assessment; then 2 sessions 2 weeks apart; then final group after 1 month follow-up assessments.	Support group: 15, 2-hour weekly psychoeducational group sessions teaching cognitive coping strategies, problem-solving and identifying supports. Strong focus on behavior problems. Assessed blindly before randomization and again at 16 weeks. (N=79)
Control (N)	No counseling, complete measures at baseline, 6 and 12 months. (N=39)	Waitlist control assessed at equivalent intervals to intervention group. Later given opportunity to participate in identical groups to study. (N=11)	Referred to existing, traditional support group through Alzheimer's Association or other health care group in Quebec. (N=79)
CG outcome measures	Caregiver Burden Interview PAIS Health Utilization Questionnaire Duke Social Support Interview Indices of Coping	BDI LSIZ ECR HDLF	RMBPC ZBI STAI Inventory of Socially Supportive Behaviors 14-item Ilfeld Psychiatric symptoms Index
CG results	No significant treatment effects for distress, burden, or psychosocial adjustment.	No significant group effects on measures of psychological and social functioning. Use of emotional discharge for coping, and use of affective regulation for coping showed significant effects for training.	No treatment group differences in burden, depression, or anxiety. Significantly greater reduction in reaction to behavior disturbance for study intervention group.
CR outcome measures	Reisberg's Stages of Cognitive Decline; Barthel Index; % institutionalized within 1 year	Not evaluated.	RMBPC
CR results	18% in intervention vs. 31% in control were institutionalized within 1 year of follow-up. That all CGs who were sons were randomized to control group may confound these results.	Not evaluated.	RMBPC change, treatment vs. control: Frequency -0.07 vs. 0.12 (p=0.06) Disruptive behaviors frequency: -0.06 vs. 0.15 (p=0.08)

Study	Roberts, et al. 1999[45]	Haley, Brown & Levine 1987[46]	Heber, et al. 2003[47]
Comments	Some whose relatives were institutionalized or died prior to follow-up measures completed questionnaires, others did not. Dropouts indicated more psychological distress at baseline.	Participants not referred for distress, levels of baseline distress highly variable across participants.	Excluded from final analyses 1 CG whose CR had died (1% of control group) and CGs whose CR had been institutionalized (15% of treatment group; 18% of controls)

Abbreviations: BDI = Beck Depression Inventory; CG = caregiver; CR = care recipient; ECR = Elderly Caregiver Family Relationship; GQ-SR = good-quality systematic review; HDLF = Health and Daily Living Form; LSIZ = Life Satisfaction Index; PAIS = Psychological Adjustment to Relative's Illness; RMBPC = Revised Memory and Behavior Problem Checklist; STAI = State Trait Anxiety Disorder; ZBI = Zarit Burden Interview.

Table 5b. RCTs of combined individual counseling and support group for caregivers of individuals with dementia

Study	Mittelman, et al. 2004 (NYU Caregiver Intervention) [42, 44, 49]	Mittelman, et al. 1995[43] Mittelman, et al. 1996[41]	Zarit, Anthony, & Boutselis 1987[48]
Population (N)	Spouse CGs of home-dwelling individuals with Alzheimer's disease, naming one additional relative in area. (N=406, with 223 completing 5 year follow-up)	Spouses of community-dwelling individual with diagnosis of Alzheimer's dementia, naming additional relative in area. (N=206)	Family member primary CG of individuals with dementia. (N=184 initial assessment, 119 completed)
Intervention (N)	Six sessions of individual and family counseling, weekly support groups after 4 months with availability of crisis counseling as needed. Topics individually determined, include BMT, support, enhancing communication. Interviewed every 4 months 1st year, then every 6 months until 2 years after death of CR or refusal. (N=203)	Six sessions of individual and family counseling, weekly support groups after 4 months with availability of crisis counseling as needed. Topics individually determined, include BMT, support, enhancing communication. Interviewed every 4 months 1st year, then every 6 months until 2 years after death of CR or refusal. (N=103)	1) Support group, 8 weekly sessions providing information about disease, problem-solving, BMT, identifying supports. (N=44) 2) Individual and family counseling, same format as above but individually and family-focused. (N=36)
Control (N)	Usual care at NYU Alzheimer's Disease Center (N=203)	Usual care at NYU Alzheimer's Disease Center (N=103)	Wait-list control assigned to intervention after 8 weeks with follow-up evaluation; post-treatment data included in assessment of effects at 1 year. (N=39)
CG outcome measures	GDRS Self-rated health assessed using a questionnaire adapted from OARS	1995: GDRS MBPC Stokes Social Networks Scale Test adapted from OARS FACES III Questionnaire 1996: Kaplan- Meier survival analysis Older Americans Resources and Service questionnaire Geriatric Depression Scale MBPC	Changes in CG's reports of stress; improvement in management of CR's problem behaviors; increased use of social support; CG's perception of treatment benefits. Revised Burden Interview BSI MBPC Caregiver Change Interview
CG results	Significantly greater change on depression measure in intervention group compared to usual care with intervention group improving. Significant treatment group effects of lower depression scores maintained through year 3 of study. Self-rated health was significantly better in the treatment group during the first 2 years of follow-up.	Intervention group significantly less depressed at 8 month measure (Mittelman 1995).	All groups, including control, reported subjective improvement, lower burden, and lower psychiatric symptoms over time, no significant group effects.
CR outcome measures	Time to nursing home placement. GDS measured but analyzed as a covariate only.	1996: GDRS Time to institutionalization	Not evaluated.

Study	Mittelman, et al. 2004 (NYU Caregiver Intervention) [42, 44, 49]	Mittelman, et al. 1995[43] Mittelman, et al. 1996[41]	Zarit, Anthony, & Boutselis 1987[48]
CR results	28.3% reduction in nursing home placement with Tx compared with control dyads (adjusted HR=0.717, p=0.025). Reduction in time from baseline to nursing home placement was 557 days: usual care = 1,209 days; enhanced counseling and support group = 1,766 days (model-predicted median).	Median length of stay at home from baseline was significantly longer for treatment group. Risk of institutionalization lower for intervention group, particularly for mild-moderate dementia.	Not evaluated.
Comments	Baseline depression significantly lower in treatment group. Used ITT analysis. Results robust across CG gender and severity of dementia. Unblinded counselors conducted follow-up assessments.	Used ITT analysis.	High attrition after first assessment (36%) attributed to family members' expressed disappointment that intervention was focused on them, not cure or help for CR.

Abbreviations: BMT = behavior management training; BSI = Brief Symptom Inventory; CG = caregiver; CR = care recipient; GDS = Global Deterioration Scale; GDRS = Geriatric Depression Rating Scale; GQ-SR = good-quality systematic review; HR = hazard ratio; ITT = intention-to-treat; MBPC = Memory and Behavior Problems Checklist; NYU = New York University; OARS = Older Americans Resource and Services Multidimensional Functional Assessment Questionnaire.

Columns separated by a dashed line indicate that the two publications appear to be related and may be based on the same study.

WIDELY CITED PSYCHOSOCIAL INTERVENTION STUDIES THAT WERE EXCLUDED FROM THIS REVIEW

We reviewed a total of 78 primary studies gleaned from 11 systematic reviews for this evidence synthesis. We excluded 48 studies when: they were not RCTs (N = 12); sample size was less than 50 (N = 23); not enough information was supplied to quality rate (3); they had group differences at baseline (1), and/or they had differential loss to follow-up (1).

Six of the 48 excluded studies have been cited frequently, occurring in five or six of the 11 systematic reviews. These six studies used a variety of interventions and reported mixed results. One study (N=36 CGs) used a six-week behavioral intervention for sleep problems and found significant improvements in sleep patterns at three-month follow-up, but no effects on CG mood or burden.[50] Another study provided counseling and information about psychological and practical home-based techniques, such as orientation and memory management strategies, to 30 patients with newly diagnosed dementia and their families. At 18-month follow-up, depression and anxiety had increased among CGs in the control group but not in the treatment group, and more CRs in the control group had been institutionalized compared with the treatment group.[51] An RCT (N=41 CGs) of a structured support group that held two-hour sessions weekly for eight weeks found no effects on CG mood or burden.[52] A study that provided CG education, stress management, and coping skills training in 14 sessions over 28 weeks reported significant reductions in CR behavioral disturbance in the intervention group (N=14), and significant CG reductions in depression in the intervention group compared with controls (N=28).[53] An eight-week intervention RCT (N=35 CGs) that compared a skills-training cognitive-behavioral group intervention to a support group that emphasized information-giving and social exchanges found no differences in CG burden or psychological distress.[54]

TECHNOLOGY-BASED INTERVENTIONS

Summary impact of technology-based interventions: There is insufficient evidence from controlled empirical studies on the effectiveness of technology-based interventions. Uncontrolled studies suggest that GPS location systems for wandering behavior may improve patient function and safety as well as reduce CG depression, burden, and stress. Robust trials with sufficient follow-up are needed to determine the feasibility, effectiveness, and cost-effectiveness of ICT interventions.

Three systematic reviews assessed the effectiveness of networked information and communications technology (ICT) interventions in supporting CGs, and included studies published through 2005,[55] 2006,[56] and 2007.[57] Although two reviews[56, 57] were largely descriptive and did not appraise the quality of the included studies, because they provided a comprehensive overview of ICT services available for individuals with dementia and their CGs, we included them in this review.

One review[57] included 15 papers that described five interventions: 1) COMPUTERLINK, a non-internet based computer network with an unmoderated forum that offers e-mail, an electronic encyclopedia, anonymous question and answers to a nurse moderator, and a decision support module; 2) Telephone-Linked Care (TLC), a computer-mediated automated telephone support system that offers automated CG stress-monitoring and counseling information, message and bulletin board support group, and a respite call for CGs; 3) Computer-Telephone Integration System (CTIS), a computerized system using Spanish and English text and voice screen phones to facilitate messaging, local information access, and support group calls; 4) AlzOnline, which offers an Internet library, message board, expert forum, and web- and telephone-based education classes; and 5) Caring for Others, an Internet-based and group videoconferencing discussion forum. The TLC and CTIS interventions were part of the REACH study.[58] The studies were RCTs of six to 18 months duration, except for one study that used a single-group pre/post-test design to evaluate the AlzOnline intervention. The sample sizes in each study ranged from 21 to 77 per group, and the comparator interventions varied in each study from no intervention, minimal support, information booklets, and family therapy. The reviewers noted that the interventions provided benefits to stress and depression for some but not all CGs, and that intervention usage varied between studies and was generally low.[57] The lack of quality appraisal of included studies was a limitation in this review.

A meta-analysis[55] combined three RCTs to determine the pooled effect of the COMPUTERLINK,[59] TLC,[58] and CTIS[60] interventions on CG depression. Although increases in subjective measures of social support, knowledge, decision-making confidence, and mental health were observed among the studies, the meta-analysis showed no significant overall effect of the technology-based interventions on depression. Heterogeneity in the types of interventions and comparators make it difficult to combine the findings across studies. The reviewers assessed the methodological quality of included studies and found that the overall quality was poor, citing unclear methods for randomization; lack of blinding; and potential for selection bias.[55]

A descriptive review of ICT-based services identified four websites and 20 publications that addressed the needs of CRs and CGs with regard to symptoms.[56] The interventions included multimedia support programs for CGs delivered via Internet, and telecare devices such as videophones to facilitate communication between CGs and healthcare providers. Interventions directed at the CR included devices and applications such as memory aids that provide reminders for daily tasks and medicine. The evidence consisted largely of case studies and small (n<50) pre- and post-test/post-test only studies, although there was one large RCT (n=299) of a multimedia Internet-based support program that provided text material and videos that modeled positive caregiving strategies. The RCT found significant improvement after 30 days in CG depression, anxiety, strain, stress, self-efficacy, intention to seek help, and perception of positive aspects of caregiving.[61] Uncontrolled studies of electronic memory aids for the CR and other assistive technologies reported improvements in carrying out daily activities and reductions of everyday memory and planning failures, suggesting the potential for such devices to support independence in the CR and reduce CG burden.

This review also identified 13 interventions that focused largely on wandering behaviors.[56] Devices included GPS-location systems; boundary alarms activated by wristband; floor-lighting systems activated upon wandering detection; communication systems instructing the patient to return to bed after failure to return for a pre-defined period of time; cooking monitoring systems; and alarms alerting the CG of wandering behavior. The evidence consisted of case studies, cross-sectional studies, or single-group, pre- and post-test/post-test only studies, and the settings included residential homes, nursing homes, and hospital settings. As one example, the Safe House Project used a single-group, post-test study of 19 families to evaluate a web-based monitoring system that included power, water, and door sensors as well as cameras. Fourteen out of 16 CGs in this study reported that the "system made life easier (e.g., peace of mind; added security; easier to keep track of individual with dementia)" and 11 out of 16 reported that "the system positively changed how the CG spends his/her time, e.g., more free time and more time for self."[62] The devices in other studies were generally found to be effective, reliable, and successful in detecting wandering, locating lost patients, and reducing patient and CG stress. More rigorous trials are needed to assess the feasibility and effectiveness of these devices in broader use within VA.

Limitations of the literature: Although there is potential for some assistive technology devices to reduce CG burden by improving the independent function of the patient and by increasing patient safety, the interventions included in these reviews were generally limited in design by the lack of a control group. Heterogeneity in the types of interventions makes it difficult to combine the findings across studies.

RESPITE CARE

Summary impact of respite care: Although a systematic review of respite care found small, statistically-significant improvements on some outcome measures, the evidence on how respite affects the health and well-being of CGs was inconsistent. Institutional/overnight respite promoted better sleep patterns in CGs during the period of respite; but there were no marked improvements in health and well-being in comparison to control groups, or compared to CG's baseline state associated with respite services of any form. The vast majority of CGs, however, frequently expressed high levels of satisfaction, and generally felt that respite services brought them various benefits, despite little evidence of significant or sustained reductions in measures of stress, depression, and burden. Many studies reported CGs' beliefs that respite enabled them to continue caring. Day care services were best studied, and the evidence for benefit for CGs and CRs was mixed. Time freed up by day care did not necessarily reduce the total amount spent on caregiving.

A 2004 systematic review compiled for the UK National Coordinating Center for NHSNHS Delivery and Organization Research & Development reviewed the effectiveness and cost-effectiveness of respite services for CGs of people with dementia.[63] The review identified 45 articles published from 1985 through 2003 that reported results on several forms of respite services. Fifteen of the 45 studies were conducted in the US, and 16 were conducted in the UK. The remaining studies were conducted in Europe (n=8), Canada (n=4), and Australia (n=2). Day care was the intervention most frequently studied.

The review examined the following outcomes:

1) Effectiveness in relation to CG's health and well-being
2) Effectiveness in relation to CRs' health, well-being, and dementia-related symptoms
3) Impact on the use of other services
4) Cost-effectiveness in relation to CG's and CRs' health and well-being

Given the comprehensive and in-depth nature of the NHS evaluation, we quote findings directly from the NHS report on the effectiveness of each type of respite care, including cost-effectiveness when evidence was available. In this report we refer to the findings on four forms of respite care that are available or might be feasible to provide in VA:

1) Day care – planned services provided outside of the home, not involving overnight stays
2) In-home respite services – involves a paid care worker coming into the family home to "sit" with the care recipient
3) Institutional/overnight respite – allows breaks away from the family home for the CR for one or more nights
4) Video respite – uses a tailored video to occupy the CR's attention, thus freeing up the CG's time for a mini-break

DAY CARE SERVICES

The NHS report identified 21 studies on day care services. Below is the summary of findings on day care services:

"Many CGs placed a high value on day care services, perceiving benefits for both themselves and the person with dementia. However, problems relating to day care attendance (e.g., lack of transportation, or the experience/belief that the patient became more confused when moved from home) acted as barriers to usage for some CGs. Few studies attempted to collect the views of people with dementia themselves, but there was some evidence to suggest patients enjoy the company, the sense of belonging and the activities provided. The evidence about the impact on CGs of using day care was unclear. Some studies showed demonstrable improvements in physical health, stress and psychological well-being, yet others showed no change. The evidence about the impact on people with dementia of day care attendance was unclear. Some studies showed improvements or stabilization, whereas others showed no positive effects. The mixed results are likely to reflect issues such as: weaknesses/differences in study design; the wide range of outcome measured used; study timescales; differences and/or deterioration in disease severity; differences in the frequency and amount of day care used. Time freed up by day care did not necessarily reduce the total amount spent on caregiving. There was some evidence to suggest that day care attendance might have a preventative effect on entry to long-term care. Two of four economic evaluations suggested that day care might be cost-saving, whereas the other half suggested that day care might provide greater benefits but at a higher cost as compared to standard care. All four studies suggested that the benefits of day care might be similar or greater than those achieved through standard care."[63]

IN-HOME RESPITE

The NHS report identified eight studies on in-home respite services. The studies used a variety of methods and considered different types of outcomes. The in-home visits typically lasted three to four hours at most, and the maximum number of hours in a given week was 19, although most services provided fewer hours. Three of the studies examined how CGs used their time during periods of in-home respite, and found little evidence that CGs used the break to engage in social or recreational activities. Instead, CGs usually did shopping or other chores; men often used the free hours to do paid work; and some CGs used the respite time for additional help with caring tasks such as lifting, bathing, and other personal hygiene tasks. One study compared in-home respite and day care on how CGs used their time. CGs spent less time on caregiving on respite days than on non-respite days with in-home respite care, whereas day care users spent more time caregiving on respite days than on non-respite days, probably in preparing the CR for going to the day care center.[63]

Below is a summary of the findings on in-home respite care:

"Carers reported high levels of satisfaction with in-home respite services. Satisfaction appeared to be closely linked to their perceptions of the benefits that the service bought to their relative, and the quality of care provided. Carers reported that they would have liked the service more often, and liked visits to last longer as the relatively short periods of respite constrained the type of activity that could be undertaken.

"None of the studies were able to demonstrate statistically significant positive effects of in-home respite on a range of measures. The evidence suggested that in-home respite could assist in maintaining family routines, and roles, and the dementia sufferer's sense of self.

"It is difficult to separate the impact of in-home respite on the demand for other types of respite care, or in reducing or delaying entry into long-term care, as most carers in these studies were accessing a range of different services.

"No evidence was retrieved in relation to the cost-effectiveness of in-home respite."[63]

INSTITUTIONAL/OVERNIGHT SERVICES
The NHS report identified 12 studies on institutional/overnight services, including two studies conducted at VA hospitals.[64, 65] One VA study assessed CG burden and depression 14 days before respite, the day of patient discharge, and 14 days post-respite, among 125 CGs whose CR had been scheduled for a two-week hospital admission for respite care. The study found transient improvement in CG burden and depression that was statistically significant at the time of discharge, but by two weeks post-respite care, these measures were not significantly different from their values two weeks prior to respite admission. Another VA study surveyed 25 CGs by telephone three days before respite admission, three days before respite discharge, and 14 days after respite discharge, and similarly found a significant reduction in psychological distress that was short-lived.[65] The lack of a control group was a limitation in these studies.

The overall findings of the NHS report on institutional/overnight respite care were as follows: "Physical and emotional benefits were seen as worthwhile when set against the difficulties of organizing institutional/overnight services. Institutional and overnight services were seen to help in some way, but other short-term breaks were seen as more beneficial to the CR. Standards of care and quality of service influence use of services. There was some evidence that CRs returned home in a worse state, but also that medical conditions could be diagnosed during breaks. Although some CGs experienced guilt in using services, others reported that services helped them to continue in their caring role. There appeared to be a major benefit to sleep, with CGs experiencing increased and better-quality sleep. There was mixed evidence on the impact of services in relation to ADL, behavior and dependency (in the CR), but it is difficult to unravel the potentially negative effects of respite from the natural progression of the disease. There was little evidence that services reduced the demand for long-term placements."[63]

Overall, there appear to be mixed benefits from institutional/overnight respite care. Sleep is improved in the CG, but the disruption to the CR's routine may be problematic. It is questionable, however, that the disease would progress enough to affect ADLs and behavior during the two-week duration, as Arksey, et al. suggests.

VIDEO RESPITE

The evidence on video respite compiled by the HTA report[63] is based on two studies by the same investigators.[66, 67] In both studies a videotape was for general viewing by persons with dementia, rather than customized for individuals, although separate tapes were made for men, women, and people from African-American, Jewish, and Hispanic backgrounds. The purpose of the videotape was to capture the CR's attention to a degree that would provide respite for the CG. In the first study, the video consisted of a 33-minute tape recorded by an actor/actress who speaks to the demented viewer, tells short stories, sings songs, and asks questions about specific subjects such as favorite activities, music, and holidays. The study found that most of the viewers with dementia remained seated and were paying attention and verbally responding throughout the viewing time.[66] The second study examined whether there was a difference in how 12 individuals with Alzheimer's watched a 20-minute videotape in a group setting compared to viewing it alone, and found that there was greater participation and response to "requests" made on the tape in a solitary setting compared with a group setting, although in both settings, viewers demonstrated at least moderate levels of interest and enjoyment.[67] There was no evidence on the effects of video respite on CG burden or CR outcomes.

Limitations of the literature: Most of the studies were not based on RCT design, and in some studies no control group was used. A number of different instruments were used to measure outcomes in the studies, and there is a wide range of intended consequences of respite care and short-term breaks. In some instances the purpose may be to assist CGs to "let go" and allow their relative to enter long-term care, while in other cases, the goal might be to support CGs to actively provide care for longer. The impact of an intervention might be difficult to capture due to the magnitude of the effect and the number of effects possible. There is a great deal of heterogeneity in this body of literature.

RECENT AND ONGOING RESEARCH STUDIES

In response to our e-mail solicitation to VA researchers and listservs, authors of unpublished and recently published studies shared with us the following findings:

- A six-month feasibility study of implementing the REACH VA intervention among 24 home-based primary care (HBPC) programs in the VHA system found decreases in CG burden, depression, and time spent in caregiving; as well as decreases in CR behavior problems. REACH VA is based on the National Institute on Aging/National Institute of Nursing Research (NIA/NINR) funded REACH II study, and provides CG support and skills training in safety, behavior management, and self-care via 12 in-home and telephone sessions, and five telephone support group sessions. The analysis found that the VHA costs of delivering the full intervention would be $2.93 per day over six months, and that satisfaction and perception of benefit from the intervention were high among both staff and CGs.[68]

- Partners in Dementia Care (PDC) is an ongoing HSR&D funded intervention that is a collaboration between local VA medical centers and Alzheimer's Association chapters. The intervention is delivered by care coordinators from each partner organization and includes a shared patient and CG assessment and ongoing action plan. PDC tests a phone-based Care Coordination Intervention that uses coaching, empowerment, and a consumer-directed approach when working with Veterans and family CGs. The Intervention assists with 1) accessing services and informal support, 2) providing information and education about dementia and caregiving, and 3) providing emotional support. The study of over 500 Veterans is in the data analysis phase, and will compare psychosocial outcomes for patients and CGs and Veteran health service use across intervention and control settings.[69]

- REACH OUT, a condensed version of the REACH II intervention that included four home visits and three phone calls over four months, was found to be feasible for use by social service agency personnel. The intervention was delivered to 272 dementia CGs, and improvements were seen in CG subjective burden, mood, social support, and health; and also in CR mood and behavior problems.[70]

- An uncontrolled pilot study of the TLC screen program examined user satisfaction and changes in CG burden, health care utilization, and costs after 12 months. The TLC program included a screen-telephone system that provided access to education, support, monitoring, and various VHA resources; as well as personal assistance from a nurse care coordinator and a support person. The study included 113 CGs of individuals with dementia. There were no significant changes after 12 months in CG outcomes including burden, depression, and ability to cope, although decreases in facility costs, hospital admissions, and hospital days of care were noted. CGs indicated that they were more satisfied with the care-coordination aspect of the program compared with the education or the monitoring.[71]

- Pilot evaluations are currently underway to determine effects on CG burden and well-being of using remote sensor technology to monitor Veterans in the HBPC program. The technology would be used to convey information about the CR's daily activities to both the CR and CG, as well as the HBPC nurse. Another ongoing study by the same investigator will determine the effects of an online Long Term Care (LTC) Resource Guide and Shared Decision Making Tool on CG well-being and LTC knowledge.[72]

- A recently completed RCT of the Telehealth Education Program, a telephone based education and support group designed for CGs of Veterans with dementia, found short-term savings in health care costs, despite that there were no significant effects on CG burden.[73]

- A proposed RCT of Preventing Aggressive Behavior in Demented Patients (PAVeD), a six- to eight-session, home-based psychoeducational intervention for individuals with dementia and pain and their CGs. The (PAVeD) intervention aims to prevent the development of aggression in demented individuals with pain. The intervention addresses the recognition and treatment of pain in the CR, increasing pleasant activities, and improving patient-caregiver communication.[69]

- A recently completed study of the Stress-Busting Program (SBP) for Family Caregivers found improvements in CG health, social function, anxiety, anger/hostility, depression, perceived stress, and burden over the course of the two-month intervention and at two and four months post-intervention. This was measured by questionnaires, biofeedback techniques, and blood assays. The study included 202 CGs of individuals with Alzheimer Disease and Related Disorders (ADRD). The intervention involved psychoeducational support groups that met 1½ hours per week for nine weeks, and stress management techniques were also taught during the sessions. In post-intervention interviews, CGs reported that the relaxation and stress management techniques enabled them to manage stress more effectively. CGs also expressed that the interaction and companionship with other CGs was a beneficial aspect of the program. CGs who completed the SBP commonly expressed that the interaction and companionship with other CGs was the most beneficial aspect of the program. CGs also reported that the relaxation and stress management techniques enabled them to manage stress more effectively.[74]

- An ongoing project entitled CARE-Plus includes CGs within the community and the VA system, and randomizes CGs to one of three groups: a psychoeducational control group, a multi-component group designed to teach specific skills to manage neuropsychiatric symptoms, and a third group that receives the multi-component intervention as well as additional self-efficacy enhancing techniques. A telehealth approach for use by home-based CGs, combined with initial and booster home visits, would be a potential application for the intervention in the VA system.[75]

KEY QUESTION #2. What are adverse effects of CG interventions?

The systematic review of respite care[63] found evidence in one study[76] to suggest that CGs using day care service actually spend more time on caregiving activities on respite days than on non-respite days, usually in preparing the CR for the visit or transporting the CR to the day care setting.

In studies of institutional/overnight respite, some CGs reported that the respite break had adversely affected the CRs, and that the disruption to their routine had increased anxiety and confusion.[63] In one study,[77] some CGs reported an increase in short-term workload because the CR's continence worsened on return home, whereas other CGs reported a loss of mobility for the CR because wheelchair use by the services had created a dependency. Another drawback identified by CGs in this study was a concern about standards of care, and 10% of the sample (n=167) who tried institutional/overnight breaks decided not to use the service again based on quality of service. In a small (n=25) study of institutional/overnight respite services, over half of CGs reported feeling sad or lonely while the patient was in the hospital, and one-fifth felt guilty and reported criticism from friends and relatives for allowing relief admission.[78]

We found no evidence of adverse effects from other CG interventions based on the systematic reviews yielded by our search, and the primary studies on psychosocial interventions we examined.

DISCUSSION

We conducted a critical assessment of systematic reviews and recently published studies on interventions for dementia CGs. We identified several promising interventions, but there was considerable variability in outcomes evaluated across interventions, and no single type of intervention was unequivocally effective on any given outcome of interest. Though the body of evidence for most interventions was limited, the following points highlight potentially promising approaches:

- The evidence on how respite affects the health and well-being of CGs is inconsistent, but respite care appears to be valued by CGs and may offer them short term benefits. Institutional/overnight respite promoted better sleep patterns in CGs during the period of respite, although there were no marked improvements in health and well-being in comparison to control groups. Short term respite care, however, may be more burdensome than beneficial for the dyad in terms of effort, preparation time, and disruption to routine.

- ICT interventions, such as GPS-location systems for wandering behavior, may improve patient function and safety as well as reduce CG burden, although current evidence is based largely on uncontrolled studies.

- Although findings were inconsistent, a limited body of evidence suggests that BMT may enhance CG well-being, depression and burden, and CR quality of life, particularly when BMT is augmented by increasing CR exercise or CG self-care behaviors.

- Individual skills training showed benefit in some studies. CG depression was ameliorated in two studies, although there were no effects on other measures of CG burden. In two other studies, disruptive behavior in the CR appeared to diminish when CGs received structured training to identify behavioral triggers and to modify the environment to reduce stress.

- CG depression may improve with both group and combined individual/group skills training interventions, particularly when the interventions are individualized by in-home assessment and targeted to specific needs of the patient-CG dyad. Ancillary improvements in positive interactions and nurturing, reducing aversive and hostile CG responses to problem behaviors, reducing CG burden, and increasing CG self-efficacy are supported by single studies.

- CG depression may respond to treatments that offer a combination of individualized counseling and group support to the CG. The combined individual/group approach also resulted in delayed institutionalization for the CR in one study. These findings are supported by a series of publications by Mittelman and colleagues, and would be strengthened by replication elsewhere. Ancillary improvements in affective regulation for coping and aversive reaction to CR behavior disturbance were supported in single studies. The effects of individual counseling and group support may vary with the skill level of the trainer, the setting, frequency and duration of contacts, and the training materials used.

- Combined exercise for CR and BMT for the CG may improve physical health and mood for the CR, although impact on CG burden, mood, quality of life, and delay of CR institutionalization has not been demonstrated.

- Supportive CG counseling based on individual assessment appears to have robust positive effects on the rate of institutionalization of the CR and on CG depression, maintained as long as three years into follow-up.

- Overall, the strongest support appears for multicomponent interventions that are designed after individual in-home assessment and tailored to the specific needs of the CG/CR dyad. Improvements in CG confidence in caregiving skills, well-being, sense of burden, stress, and mood can be seen with combined approaches. Although there is no clear evidence that institutionalization of the CR may be delayed, it does appear that behavioral symptoms of dementia can be reduced through multicomponent interventions for at least four months after intervention, and this likely improves the home atmosphere for both CR and CG.

The feasibility of implementation and cost analyses of these interventions need to be assessed within VA. Individualized programs may be the most effective but would require more resources of staff to evaluate the dyad and generate a tailored program. One cost benefit analysis of the REACH II multicomponent intervention in Memphis, Tennessee[79] indicated that training in dementia problem areas, behavior management techniques, and supportive contact can result in sparing dementia CGs an hour a day from caregiving tasks, at an estimated cost of $5 per day.

Loss to follow up appeared problematic for many of the studies in this review, and may be clinically important. This may highlight issues of intervention acceptability to dementia CGs, and reasons for dropout should be assessed and help guide future implementation efforts in this field.

We noted inconsistent and sometimes disappointing findings among the variety of interventions for dementia CGs. For example, the lack of effect for respite care in reducing CG burden and premature CR institutionalization seems intuitively surprising. It is possible that the relentless decline and challenge of dementia poses a stable negative impact that overwhelms more transient improvements in mood, burden, quality of life, and support for maintaining CRs in the home. This may indicate that the definition of what constitutes meaningful change in this field and whether the instruments used are sensitive enough to detect it need to be reevaluated.

Alternatively, the measures used to define the psychosocial outcomes of depression, burden, coping, quality of life, and CR behavior problems as constructs may lack adequate sensitivity to detect meaningful change in the context of dementia. For example, across the 30 primary studies reported here, the Center for Epidemiologic Studies Depression Scale (CES-D) was used to measure depression in nine studies, and one-third of those studies reported a significant reduction in CG depression in the intervention group. It is possible that the benefits of the interventions employed in the studies were important to the CGs but too subtle to result in enduring change on the CES-D. We attempted to examine the performance of measures for CG depression, burden, and CR behavior problems across the 37 studies reviewed here, but the samples were too small to derive strong conclusions about whether specific measures were more likely to detect improvements. Only four measures were used in six or more studies; they were associated with a study reporting significant improvement from baseline among CGs in the following proportions: Geriatric Depression Rating Scale 43%; CES-D 33%; Zarit Burden Inventory 17%; Memory and Behavior Problems Checklist (MBPC) or Revised Memory and Behavior Problems Checklist (RMBPC) 33%. As early as 1987, Zarit, et al. wrote that global ratings of distress and burden may not reflect the changes or possible benefits that CGs may be experiencing, yet these measures continue to be used widely.

The evidence on psychosocial interventions is limited by differences in the interventions used across studies. Furthermore, many studies assessed complex interventions and it was difficult to determine with confidence which aspect of the intervention was effective. However, the addition of the REACH studies following expert panel commentary increased the perspective of this review, and may suggest that the specific intervention or combination of interventions is not as important as the role of individual assessment and tailoring of interventions to the needs of the dyad through multiple modalities. Viewed through this lens, intervention variability and adaptability may be an important feature of a successful intervention, permitting responsiveness to variation across individuals.

There was potentially more compromising variations in recruitment strategies and analytic methods across studies. For example, some studies excluded from final analysis the data from CGs whose CR had died or moved to institutional care settings[47] while others did not.[80] Some studies drew from a distressed population seeking assistance where response to treatment may be more evident,[34] while others sampled from general clinic or Alzheimer's Association membership rosters.[46]

Outcome measures and interventions varied widely across studies, but complications also arise when these aspects overlap imperfectly. We had difficulty sorting the studies into discrete intervention groups, and noted, for example, that skills-based interventions often included aspects of the more precisely defined behavior management training, and that supportive counseling similarly offered components of skills training as part of the intervention. Psychosocial interventions do not lend themselves to the same precise sorting and control as a medication trial might. From published reports, it was not possible to compare adherence to therapeutic protocol, or an individual interventionist's ability to form rapport with the subjects across studies, or assess how these factors contributed to outcomes. It is likely these instrumentation issues varied considerably across studies.

A further source of discrepancy in results may stem from individual variation. Across studies, we noted a number of factors that should be controlled for in future studies and considered when weighing treatment options for CG/CR dyads in dementia. More severe CG depression at baseline can result in differential dropout and poor treatment adherence.[13, 26] Burgio, et al. report differential effects for African American CGs compared to Caucasian American CGs: a skills-training intervention was more effective for reducing bother among African American CGs, whereas minimal support phone contacts were more effective for White CGs.[38] Interventions can have different effects for spousal CGs than for nonspouses[28, 38] and for female versus male CGs.[28] Brodaty and colleagues reported they solicited from CGs which part of the program had been most useful and found "marked variety in the answers, suggesting that different components were helpful for different CGs."[6]

There were also limitations to generalizing findings from the review of technology-based interventions. The reviews were largely descriptive and did not appraise the quality of the included studies. Older systematic reviews that performed quality appraisal of RCTs contained evidence from four RCTs on phone and computer-based interventions that may no longer be relevant as technology develops. However, the studies reviewed provide a comprehensive overview of ICT services available for individuals with dementia and their CGs.

Given that the efficacy of an intervention varies with the individual, individualized multicomponent treatments may well hold the most promise. This conclusion is consistent with the pattern of findings reported in this synthesis project. We agree with the conclusions of Brodaty, et al. in their 2003 systematic review that multicomponent, individualized treatments targeting specific problems identified by the CG while offering combined individual and group interaction appear to produce the most identifiable meaningful change in CG mood and coping.[81] This conclusion is also aligned with Schulz et al.,[82] who wrote in an overview of the REACH studies that "Many caregiving interventions involve several treatment elements aimed at simultaneously addressing multiple problems. Multicomponent interventions delivered in high doses are generally more effective than more narrowly targeted interventions…[however] we believe a 'one size fits all' approach to CG interventions is likely to be ineffective" (p. 519).

This review is also limited by the dates of literature covered by the good quality systematic reviews we included. The most recent reviews included in our synthesis were published in 2009; and the most recent literature searches conducted by these reviews extended through 2007 for technology-based interventions,[57] and through 2005 for psychosocial interventions.[83] Given the broad scope of our review, we examined previous systematic reviews in search of compelling evidence of significant benefit from CG interventions. Because previous reviews and the trials they identified did not show compelling evidence of benefit in any particular intervention, we did not conduct a systematic search for recently published RCTs. To address the likelihood that newer trials published since 2007 have found strong evidence of benefit but were not considered in our review, we added newer original studies to this overall document upon the recommendation of our expert review panel. We felt the studies recommended by our expert panel represented highly regarded, well-constructed RCTs that added new strength to the literature. In fact, the quality of studies emerging from the REACH program caused us to reappraise the strength of multicomponent interventions, while studies added on recommendation also persuaded us that case management appears to be a stronger contributor to CG coping and quality of life than originally assessed. While the process of beginning with a review of reviews and then adding specific new studies recommended by expert peers may have resulted in a less systematic representation of the recent literature (published after 2006), we tried to minimize that problem by including a wide variety of experts on our panel, and also included the AoA Compendium[2] to bolster comprehensiveness.

We noted that many studies eliminated by our quality rating have been included in four, five, or even six major systematic reviews frequently cited in the field. Psychosocial studies of vulnerable populations tend to be laden with challenges from the outset, and there may be a need to use less stringent quality criteria in order to assess the contributions of the field. In order to narrow our search to the best quality data, we identified the studies that have been frequently cited, and assessed their quality using standard criteria and group consensus. This approach also has its weaknesses. There may be good quality studies reviewed in poor quality reviews that were not captured in this project. Also, subtle, transient, individual subject responses may be a more appropriate indicator of effectiveness when intervening with dementia CR/CG dyads, and current evidence synthesis conventions evaluating statistical significance may not be ideally equipped to isolate these small but potentially clinically meaningful effects.

The distinction between clinical and statistical significance is important to the topic of dementia CG interventions. Schulz and colleagues (2002) conducted a systematic review with the explicit intent of evaluating the clinical importance of outcomes for dementia CGs.[84] They required *a priori* that an effect has statistical significance before evaluating the clinical significance, which they defined by one of four indicators: 1) improvement towards normal functioning in clinical symptoms; 2) improvement in quality of life; 3) importance of an outcome to society; and 4) social validity (extent to which research participants and experts judge the interventions and outcomes to be acceptable). They concluded that psychosocial interventions appeared promising for clinically significant outcomes in CG depression, based on clinical improvements seen in two of 24 studies reviewed.[30, 85] Psychosocial interventions also appeared to be promising for targeting CG anxiety (four of seven studies showed small clinical improvements). Small positive effects were noted for CG quality of life, but the heterogeneity of interventions rendered it difficult to attribute outcomes to specific causes, and there was no overall good standard for judging what constitutes a clinically significant change in this cluster. Delay of institutionalization (an important social outcome) was clinically important in six of seven heterogeneous interventions reviewed. The authors noted that most studies met criteria for social validity, but those ratings were possibly biased as subjects may have felt obligated to report positive comments to please researchers or to justify their own challenges in participating. In sum, methods for determining clinical significance remain somewhat unstandardized, but scrutiny of dementia CG interventions reveals some promise of clinical utility for CG depression/anxiety, and evidence that outcomes of these interventions are socially important.

FUTURE RESEARCH RECOMMENDATIONS

Based on our examination of primary studies used in previous systematic reviews, CG interventions that appear to be effective tend to be individually-tailored treatments that are more resource-intensive, such as BMT and individual skills training. Our informal survey of recently completed and ongoing studies using VA e-mail listservs identified preliminary studies of psychosocial interventions (REACH OUT;[70] REACH VA;[68] Stress-Busting Program[74]) and technology-based interventions (Telehealth Education Program;[73] TLC[71]) that found improvements in CG burden with some of the interventions, and short-term savings in health care costs in one study.[73] Studies of other psychosocial interventions (PAVeD; PDC[69]) and technology-based interventions[72] have been proposed or are underway. In order to determine the feasibility of implementation, effectiveness, and cost-effectiveness of CG interventions within VA settings, future studies should evaluate different implementation strategies, evaluate interventions in different settings, and evaluate methods for improving participant retention. Given some of the methodologic weaknesses in past studies, future studies should use rigorous study designs, sufficient sample size, and appropriate duration of follow-up.

The wide range of outcomes used to evaluate the effects of CG interventions reflects the diversity in what CGs and researchers consider effective. In addition to their review of published studies on respite care, Arksey, et al.[63] conducted a qualitative consultation with multiple stakeholders, including CGs, CRs, and health and social care professionals. Key objectives of the consultation were to examine the gaps in the literature and to examine whether the outcomes that CGs value are the same as, or similar to, those used in the research literature. The contributors to the consultation generally felt that respite was too complex to be evaluated by one or two measures of effectiveness. They proposed a range of qualitative and quantitative indicators against which they felt the effectiveness of respite services should be measured. Proposed quantifiable measures included the following: 1) a comparison of the CR's health, both physical and mental, on admission and discharge, within the context of clear individual health goals; 2) a similar assessment of the health of the CG; and 3) the impact of activities/stimulation on the CR's behavior, sleep patterns, ADL, etc."[63]

Similar studies of CG perceptions with regard to other interventions would potentially offer a rich source of inspiration for the development of tools that measure what we hope to measure in this field: evidence that the CG has perceived and responded to useful intervention that improves the quality of experience within the here and now. We need to understand what interventions to offer to a CG who is depleted by months of challenging daily assistance to a loved one with dementia, and evaluate interventions that might impact those outcomes for cost and utility. Qualitative studies to identify outcomes that are important to individuals with dementia and their CGs within the VA system would serve future research and policy for promoting the best welfare of aging veterans and their community CGs.

REFERENCES

1. Veterans Health Administration Office of the Assistant Deputy Under Secretary for Health for Policy and Planning. Projections of the prevalence and incidence of dementias including Alzheimer's Disease for the total, enrolled, and patient veteran populations aged 65 or over. 2004. *http://www4.va.gov/HEALTHPOLICYPLANNING/reports1.asp*.

2. Administration on Aging's Alzheimer's Disease Supportive Services Program. Annotated Bibliography: Evidence-based interventions that target people with ADRD or their caregivers. *http://www.aoa.gov/AoARoot/AoA_Programs/HCLTC/Alz_Grants/docs/EB2010.pdf*. 2010.

3. Pinquart M, Sorensen S. Helping caregivers of persons with dementia: which interventions work and how large are their effects? *Int Psychogeriatr.* Dec 2006;18(4):577-595.

4. Harris RP, Helfand M, Woolf SH, et al. Current methods of the US Preventive Services Task Force. A review of the process. *American Journal of Preventive Medicine.* 2001;30(3S):21-35.

5. Oxman AD, Guyatt GH. Validation of an index of the quality of review articles. *J Clin Epidemiol.* 1991;44(11):1271-1278.

6. Brodaty H, Gresham M, Luscombe G. The Prince Henry Hospital dementia caregivers' training programme. *Int J Geriatr Psychiatry.* Feb 1997;12(2):183-192.

7. Folstein MF, Folstein SE, McHugh PR. "Mini-mental state". A practical method for grading the cognitive state of patients for the clinician. *J Psychiatr Res.* Nov 1975;12(3):189-198.

8. Hughes CP, Berg L, Danziger WL, Coben LA, Martin RL. A new clinical scale for the staging of dementia. *Br J Psychiatry.* Jun 1982;140:566-572.

9. Drummond MF, Mohide EA, Tew M, Streiner DL, Pringle DM, Gilbert JR. Economic evaluation of a support program for caregivers of demented elderly. *Int J Technol Assess Health Care.* 1991;7(2):209-219.

10. Belle SH, Burgio L, Burns R, et al. Enhancing the quality of life of dementia caregivers from different ethnic or racial groups: a randomized, controlled trial.[Summary for patients in Ann Intern Med. 2006 Nov 21;145(10):I39; PMID: 17116914]. *Ann Intern Med.* Nov 21 2006;145(10):727-738.

11. Holland JM, Currier JM, Gallagher-Thompson D, Holland JM, Currier JM, Gallagher-Thompson D. Outcomes from the Resources for Enhancing Alzheimer's Caregiver Health (REACH) program for bereaved caregivers. *Psychology & Aging.* Mar 2009;24(1):190-202.

12. Gitlin LN, Winter L, Dennis MP, et al. A biobehavioral home-based intervention and the well-being of patients with dementia and their caregivers: the COPE randomized trial. *Jama.* Sep 1 2010;304(9):983-991.

13. Castro CM, Wilcox S, O'Sullivan P, et al. An exercise program for women who are caring for relatives with dementia. *Psychosom Med.* May-Jun 2002;64(3):458-468.

14. Callahan CM, Boustani MA, Unverzagt FW, et al. Effectiveness of collaborative care for older adults with Alzheimer disease in primary care: a randomized controlled trial. *Jama.* May 10 2006;295(18):2148-2157.

15. Vickrey BG, Mittman BS, Connor KI, et al. The effect of a disease management intervention on quality and outcomes of dementia care: a randomized, controlled trial.[Summary for patients in Ann Intern Med. 2006 Nov 21;145(10):I31; PMID: 17116913]. *Ann Intern Med.* Nov 21 2006;145(10):713-726.

16. Eloniemi-Sulkava U, Notkola IL, Hentinen M, Kivela SL, Sivenius J, Sulkava R. Effects of supporting community-living demented patients and their caregivers: a randomized trial. *Journal of the American Geriatrics Society.* Oct 2001;49(10):1282-1287.

17. Miller R, Newcomer R, Fox P. Effects of the Medicare Alzheimer's Disease Demonstration on nursing home entry. *Health Serv Res.* Aug 1999;34(3):691-714.

18. Newcomer R, Yordi C, DuNah R, Fox P, Wilkinson A. Effects of the Medicare Alzheimer's Disease Demonstration on caregiver burden and depression. *Health Serv Res.* Aug 1999;34(3):669-689.

19. Teri L, McCurry SM, Logsdon R, et al. Training community consultants to help family members improve dementia care: a randomized controlled trial. *Gerontologist.* Dec 2005;45(6):802-811.

20. Gormley N, Lyons D, Howard R. Behavioural management of aggression in dementia: a randomized controlled trial. *Age Ageing.* Mar 2001;30(2):141-145.

21. Teri L, Gibbons LE, McCurry SM, et al. Exercise plus behavioral management in patients with Alzheimer disease: a randomized controlled trial. *Jama.* Oct 15 2003;290(15):2015-2022.

22. Burns R, Nichols LO, Martindale-Adams J, et al. Primary care interventions for dementia caregivers: 2-year outcomes from the REACH study. *Gerontologist.* Aug 2003;43(4):547-555.

23. Gallagher-Thompson D, Gray HL, Tang PC, et al. Impact of in-home behavioral management versus telephone support to reduce depressive symptoms and perceived stress in Chinese caregivers: results of a pilot study. *Am J Geriatr Psychiatry.* May 2007;15(5):425-434.

24. Gonyea JG, O'Connor MK, Boyle PA, Gonyea JG, O'Connor MK, Boyle PA. Project CARE: a randomized controlled trial of a behavioral intervention group for Alzheimer's disease caregivers. *Gerontologist.* Dec 2006;46(6):827-832.

25. Farran CJ, Gilley DW, McCann JJ, et al. Efficacy of behavioral interventions for dementia caregivers. *West J Nurs Res.* Dec 2007;29(8):944-960.

26. Buckwalter KC, Gerdner L, Kohout F, et al. A nursing intervention to decrease depression in family caregivers of persons with dementia. *Arch Psychiatr Nurs.* Apr 1999;13(2):80-88.

27. Bass DM, Clark PA, Looman WJ, et al. The Cleveland Alzheimer's managed care demonstration: outcomes after 12 months of implementation. *Gerontologist.* Feb 2003;43(1):73-85.

28. Gerdner LA, Buckwalter KC, Reed D. Impact of a psychoeducational intervention on caregiver response to behavioral problems. *Nursing Research.* Nov-Dec 2002;51(6):363-374.

29. Gitlin LN, Corcoran M, Winter L, Boyce A, Hauck WW. A randomized, controlled trial of a home environmental intervention: effect on efficacy and upset in caregivers and on daily function of persons with dementia. *Gerontologist.* Feb 2001;41(1):4-14.

30. Teri L, Logsdon RG, Uomoto J, McCurry SM. Behavioral treatment of depression in dementia patients: a controlled clinical trial. *Journals of Gerontology Series B-Psychological Sciences & Social Sciences.* Jul 1997;52(4):P159-166.

31. Wright LK, Litaker M, Laraia MT, DeAndrade S. Continuum of care for Alzheimer's disease: a nurse education and counseling program. *Issues Ment Health Nurs.* Apr-May 2001;22(3):231-252.

32. Coon DW, Thompson L, Steffen A, et al. Anger and depression management: psycho-educational skill training interventions for women caregivers of a relative with dementia. *Gerontologist.* Oct 2003;43(5):678-689.

33. Corbeil RR, Quayhagen MP, Quayhagen M. Intervention effects on dementia caregiving interaction: a stress-adaptation modeling approach. *J Aging Health.* Feb 1999;11(1):79-95.

34. Hepburn KW, Tornatore J, Center B, Ostwald SW. Dementia family caregiver training: affecting beliefs about caregiving and caregiver outcomes. *Journal of the American Geriatrics Society.* Apr 2001;49(4):450-457.

35. Ostwald SK, Hepburn KW, Caron W, Burns T, Mantell R. Reducing caregiver burden: a randomized psychoeducational intervention for caregivers of persons with dementia. *Gerontologist.* Jun 1999;39(3):299-309.

36. Hepburn KW, Lewis M, Narayan S, et al. Partners in Caregiving: a psychoeducation program affecting dementia family caregivers' distress and caregiving outlook. *Clinical Gerontologist.* 2006;29(1):53-69.

37. Bourgeois MS, Schulz R, Burgio LD, Beach S. Skills training for spouses of patients with Alzheimer's Disease: outcomes of an intervention study. *Journal of Clinical Geropsychology.* 2002;8(1):53-73.

38. Burgio L, Stevens A, Guy D, et al. Impact of two psychosocial interventions on white and African American family caregivers of individuals with dementia. *Gerontologist.* Aug 2003;43(4):568-579.

39. Hepburn K, Lewis M, Tornatore J, et al. The Savvy Caregiver program: the demonstrated effectiveness of a transportable dementia caregiver psychoeducation program. *J Gerontol Nurs.* Mar 2007;33(3):30-36.

40. Hepburn KW, Lewis M, Sherman CW, et al. The savvy caregiver program: developing and testing a transportable dementia family caregiver training program. *Gerontologist.* Dec 2003;43(6):908-915.

41. Mittelman MS, Ferris SH, Shulman E, Steinberg G, Levin B. A family intervention to delay nursing home placement of patients with Alzheimer disease. A randomized controlled trial. *Jama.* Dec 4 1996;276(21):1725-1731.

42. Mittelman MS, Roth DL, Coon DW, et al. Sustained benefit of supportive intervention for depressive symptoms in caregivers of patients with Alzheimer's disease. *Am J Psychiatry.* May 2004;161(5):850-856.

43. Mittelman MS, Ferris SH, Shulman E, et al. A comprehensive support program: effect on depression in spouse-caregivers of AD patients. *Gerontologist.* Dec 1995;35(6):792-802.

44. Mittelman MS, Roth DL, Clay OJ, et al. Preserving health of Alzheimer caregivers: impact of a spouse caregiver intervention. *Am J Geriatr Psychiatry.* Sep 2007;15(9):780- 789.

45. Roberts J, Browne G, Milne C, et al. Problem-solving counseling for caregivers of the cognitively impaired: effective for whom? *Nursing Research.* May-Jun 1999;48(3):162-172.

46. Haley WE, Brown SL, Levine EG. Experimental evaluation of the effectiveness of group intervention for dementia caregivers. *Gerontologist.* Jun 1987;27(3):376-382.

47. Hebert R, Levesque L, Vezina J, et al. Efficacy of a psychoeducative group program for caregivers of demented persons living at home: a randomized controlled trial. *Journals of Gerontology Series B-Psychological Sciences & Social Sciences.* Jan 2003;58(1):S58-67.

48. Zarit SH, Anthony CR, Boutselis M. Interventions with care givers of dementia patients: comparison of two approaches. *Psychology & Aging.* Sep 1987;2(3):225-232.

49. Mittelman MS, Haley WE, Clay OJ, et al. Improving caregiver well-being delays nursing home placement of patients with Alzheimer disease. *Neurology.* Nov 14 2006;67(9):1592-1599.

50. McCurry SM, Logsdon RG, Vitiello MV, Teri L. Successful behavioral treatment for reported sleep problems in elderly caregivers of dementia patients: a controlled study. *Journals of Gerontology Series B-Psychological Sciences & Social Sciences.* Mar 1998;53(2):P122-129.

51. Moniz-Cook E, Agar S, Gibson G, Win T, Wang M. A preliminary study of the effects of early intervention with people with dementia and their families in a memory clinic. *Aging Ment Health.* 1998;2(3):199 - 211.

52. Hebert R, Leclerc G, Bravo G, Dirouard D, Lefrancois R. Efficacy of a support group programme for caregivers of demented patients in the community: a randomized controlled trial. *Archives of Gerontology and Geriatrics.* 1994;18:1-4.

53. Marriott A, Donaldson C, Tarrier N, Burns A. Effectiveness of cognitive-behavioural family intervention in reducing the burden of care in carers of patients with Alzheimer's disease. *Br J Psychiatry.* Jun 2000;176:557-562.

54. Gendron C, Poitras L, Dastoor D, Perodeau G. Cognitive-Behavioral Group Intervention for Spousal Caregivers: Findings and Clinical Considerations. *Clinical Gerontologist.* 1996;17(1):3-19.

55. Thompson CA, Spilsbury K, Hall J, Birks Y, Barnes C, Adamson J. Systematic review of information and support interventions for caregivers of people with dementia. *BMC Geriatr.* 2007;7:18.

56. Lauriks S, Reinersmann A, Van der Roest HG, et al. Review of ICT-based services for identified unmet needs in people with dementia. *Ageing Res Rev.* Oct 2007;6(3):223-246.

57. Powell J, Chiu T, Eysenbach G. A systematic review of networked technologies supporting carers of people with dementia. *J Telemed Telecare.* 2008;14(3):154-156.

58. Mahoney DF, Tarlow BJ, Jones RN. Effects of an automated telephone support system on caregiver burden and anxiety: findings from the REACH for TLC intervention study. *Gerontologist.* Aug 2003;43(4):556-567.

59. Brennan PF, Moore SM, Smyth KA. The effects of a special computer network on caregivers of persons with Alzheimer's disease. *Nursing Research.* May-Jun 1995;44(3):166-172.

60. Eisdorfer C, Czaja SJ, Loewenstein DA, et al. The effect of a family therapy and technology-based intervention on caregiver depression. *Gerontologist.* Aug 2003;43(4):521-531.

61. Beauchamp N, Irvine AB, Seeley J, et al. Worksite-based internet multimedia program for family caregivers of persons with dementia. *Gerontologist.* Dec 2005;45(6):793-801.

62. Kinney JM, Kart CS, Murdoch LD, Conley CJ. Striving to provide safety assistance for families of elders - The Safe House project. *Dementia: the international journal of social research and practice.* 2004;3(3):351-370.

63. Arksey H, Jackson K, Croucher K, et al. *Review of respite services and short-term breaks for carers for people with dementia.* London: NHS SDO; 2004.

64. Adler G, Ott L, Jelinski M, Mortimer J, Christensen R. Institutional respite care: benefits and risks for dementia patients and caregivers. *International Psychogeriatrics.* 1993;5(1):67-77.

65. Larkin JP, Hopcroft BM. In-hospital respite as a moderator of caregiver stress. *Health Soc Work.* May 1993;18(2):132-138.

66. Lund DA, Hill RD, Caserta MS, Wright SD. Video Respite: an innovative resource for family, professional caregivers, and persons with dementia. *Gerontologist.* Oct 1995;35(5):683-687.

67. Caserta MS, Lund DA. Video Respite in an Alzheimer's care center: Group versus solitary viewing. . *Activities, Adaptation & Aging.* 2002 27(1):13-28.

68. Nichols LO, Martindale-Adams J. Resources for Enhancing Alzheimer's Caregivers Health in the VA (REACH VA). *Unpublished abstract; personal communication.*

69. Kunik ME. *Personal communication.*

70. Burgio LD, Collins IB, Schmid B, et al. Translating the REACH caregiver intervention for use by area agency on aging personnel: the REACH OUT program. *Gerontologist.* Feb 2009;49(1):103-116.

71. Dang S, Remon N, Harris J, et al. Care coordination assisted by technology for multiethnic caregivers of persons with dementia: a pilot clinical demonstration project on caregiver burden and depression. *Journal of Telemedicine & Telecare.* 2008;14(8):443-447.

72. Reder S. *Personal communication.*

73. Wray LO, Shulan MD, Toseland RW, Freeman K, Vasquez BE, Gao J. The effect of telephone support groups on costs of care for Veterans with dementia. *Unpublished abstract; personal communication.*

74. Miner-Williams D. Relaxation Therapy for Alzheimer's Caregivers. *Personal communication.*

75. O'Connor MK. *Personal communication.*

76. Berry GL, Zarit SH, Rabatin VX. Caregiver activity on respite and nonrespite days: a comparison of two service approaches. *Gerontologist.* Dec 1991;31(6):830-835.

77. Levin E, Moriarty J, Gorbach P. *Better for the Break.* London: HMSO and National Institute for Social Work; 1994.

78. Pearson ND. An assessment of relief hospital admissions for elderly patients with dementia. *Health Trends.* Nov 1988;20(4):120-121.

79. Nichols LO, Chang C, Lummus A, et al. The cost-effectiveness of a behavior intervention with caregivers of patients with Alzheimer's disease. *Journal of the American Geriatrics Society.* Mar 2008;56(3):413-420.

80. Roberts J, Browne G, Gafni A, Varieur M, Loney P, De Ruijter M. Specialized continuing care models for persons with dementia: a systematic review of the research literature. *Can J Aging.* 2000;19:106-126.

81. Brodaty H, Green A, Koschera A. Meta-analysis of psychosocial interventions for caregivers of people with dementia. *Journal of the American Geriatrics Society.* May 2003;51(5):657-664.

82. Schulz R, Burgio L, Burns R, et al. Resources for Enhancing Alzheimer's Caregiver Health (REACH): overview, site-specific outcomes, and future directions. *Gerontologist.* Aug 2003;43(4):514-520.

83. Thompson CCA, Spilsbury K. Support for carers of people with Alzheimer's type dementia. *Cochrane Database of Systematic Reviews.* 2009(2).

84. Schulz R, O'Brien A, Czaja S, et al. Dementia caregiver intervention research: in search of clinical significance. *Gerontologist.* Oct 2002;42(5):589-602.

85. Gallagher-Thompson D, Lovett S, Rose J, et al. Impact of psychoeducational interventions on distressed family caregivers. *Journal of Clinical Geropsychology* 2000;6(2):91-110.

APPENDIX A. INCLUSION/EXCLUSION CRITERIA

1. Is the publication a systematic review/meta-analysis?
   a. No .... STOP ☐
   b. Yes .... ☐
   Most recent year of publication within search strategy: _____

2. Does the study population include non-professional caregivers of individuals with dementia of any severity?
   a. No .... STOP ☐
   b. Yes .... ☐

3. Did the study evaluate the effectiveness, safety, or cost of any of the following types of interventions?
   Psychoeducational interventions .... ☐
   Cognitive-behavioral interventions .... ☐
   Counseling/case-management .... ☐
   General support services .... ☐
   Respite care .... ☐
   Telephone-based support groups/education .... ☐
   Home TeleHealth/Health Buddy home monitoring device .... ☐
   Internet-based resources and caregiver assistance programs .... ☐
   Physical activity .... ☐
   Multicomponent interventions .... ☐
   Other, specify .... ☐
   None of the above .... STOP ☐

4. Does the study report on any of the following caregiver outcomes?
   Knowledge and ability to manage problematic behavior .... ☐
   Psychosocial outcomes (burden/subjective well-being, depression, anxiety, perceived self-efficacy, quality of life, etc.) .... ☐
   Health behaviors (e.g., diet, exercise, sleep) .... ☐
   Health (e.g., reported health, symptoms, medication use/misuse, service use, mortality .... ☐
   Other, specify .... ☐
   None of the above .... proceed to Q5 ☐

5. Does the study report on any of the following patient outcomes?
   Use of psychotropic drugs .... ☐
   Cognition .... ☐
   Mood .... ☐
   Behavioral disturbances .... ☐
   Social function .... ☐
   Physical function .... ☐
   Hospitalizations, institutionalization, or other health care visits, including ER visits .... ☐
   Accidents .... ☐
   Health-related quality of life .... ☐
   Satisfaction with health care .... ☐
   Other, specify .... ☐
   None of the above .... proceed to Q6 ☐

6. Is the text of the article in English?
   a. No .... ☐
   b. Yes .... ☐

7. If this article meets no other criterion, should it be saved for background or discussion?
   a. No .... STOP ☐
   b. Yes: narrative review with potentially useful references .... STOP ☐
   c. Yes: primary study, possibly more recent than existing SRs .... ☐
   d. Yes: clinical guidelines .... ☐
   e. Yes: other, specify .... ☐

Key words, notes:	Full text code:

APPENDIX B. QUALITY RATING CRITERIA FOR SYSTEMATIC REVIEWS*

Overall quality rating for each systematic review is based on the below questions. Ratings are summarized as: *Good, Fair, or Poor*:

- Search dates reported? *Yes or No*
- Search methods reported? *Yes or No*
- Comprehensive search? *Yes or No*
- Inclusion criteria reported? *Yes or No*
- Selection bias avoided? *Yes or No*
- Validity criteria reported? *Yes or No*
- Validity assessed appropriately? *Yes or No*
- Methods used to combine studies reported? *Yes or No*
- Findings combined appropriately? *Yes or No*
- Conclusions supported by data? *Yes or No*

Definitions of ratings based on above criteria

Good: Meets all criteria: Reports comprehensive and reproducible search methods and results; reports pre-defined criteria to select studies and reports reasons for excluding potentially relevant studies; adequately evaluates quality of included studies and incorporates assessments of quality when synthesizing data; reports methods for synthesizing data and uses appropriate methods to combine data qualitatively or quantitatively; and conclusions supported by the evidence reviewed.

Fair: Studies will be graded fair if they fail to meet one or more of the above criteria, but the limitations are not judged as being major.

Poor: Studies will be graded poor if they have a major limitation in one or more of the above criteria.

*Based on the following publications:

Harris RP, Helfand M, Woolf SH, et al. Current methods of the US Preventive Services Task Force: a review of the process. *Am J Prev Med.* 2001:20(3S); 21-35.

National Institute for Health and Clinical Excellence. The Guidelines Manual. London: Institute for Health and Clinical Excellence; 2006.

Oxman AD, Guyatt GH. Validation of an index of the quality of review articles. *J Clin Epidemiol.* 1991;44:1271-8.

APPENDIX C.   USPSTF QUALITY RATING CRITERIA FOR RANDOMIZED CONTROLLED TRIALS (RCTS) AND COHORT STUDIES

CRITERIA

- Initial assembly of comparable groups: RCTs—adequate randomization, including concealment and whether potential confounders were distributed equally among groups; cohort studies—consideration of potential confounders with either restriction or measurement for adjustment in the analysis; consideration of inception cohorts

- Maintenance of comparable groups (includes attrition, cross-overs, adherence, contamination)

- Important differential loss to follow-up or overall high loss to follow-up

- Measurements: equal, reliable, and valid (includes masking of outcome assessment)

- Clear definition of interventions

- Important outcomes considered

- Analysis: adjustment for potential confounders for cohort studies, or intention-to-treat analysis for RCTs (i.e. analysis in which all participants in a trial are analyzed according to the intervention to which they were allocated, regardless of whether or not they completed the intervention)

Definition of ratings based on above criteria

Good: Meets all criteria: Comparable groups are assembled initially and maintained throughout the study (follow-up at least 80 percent); reliable and valid measurement instruments are used and applied equally to the groups; interventions are spelled out clearly; important outcomes are considered; and appropriate attention to confounders in analysis.

Fair: Studies will be graded "fair" if any or all of the following problems occur, without the important limitations noted in the "poor" category below: Generally comparable groups are assembled initially but some question remains whether some (although not major) differences occurred in follow-up; measurement instruments are acceptable (although not the best) and generally applied equally; some but not all important outcomes are considered; and some but not all potential confounders are accounted for.

Poor: Studies will be graded "poor" if any of the following major limitations exists: Groups assembled initially are not close to being comparable or maintained throughout the study; unreliable or invalid measurement instruments are used or not applied at all equally among groups (including not masking outcome assessment); and key confounders are given little or no attention.

APPENDIX D. ABBREVIATIONS

AA	African American
AD	Alzheimer's Disease
ADL	Activities of daily living
ADRDA	Alzheimer Disease and Related Disorders Association
AHRQ	Agency for Healthcare Research and Quality
AoA	Administration on Aging
BACS	Beliefs about Caregiving Scale
BDI	Beck Depression Inventory
BDRS	Blessed Dementia Rating Scale
BEHAVE	Behavioral Pathology in Alzheimer's Disease Rating Scale
BMT	Behavior management training
CES-D	Center for Epidemiologic Studies Depression Scale
CG	Caregiver
CMIA	Cohen-Mansfield Agitation Inventory
CI	Confidence interval
COPE	Care of Persons with Dementia in their Environments
CQLI	Caregiver Quality of Life Instrument
CR	Care recipient
CSDD	Cornell Scale for Depression in Dementia
CTIS	Computer-Telephone Integration System
DRS	Depression Rating Scale
DSC	Dementia Steering Committee
ECR	Elderly Caregiver Family Relationship
EPC	Evidence Based Practice Center
ESP	Evidence-based Synthesis Program
FIM	Functional Independence Measure
GDRS	Geriatric Depression Rating Scale
GDS	Global Deterioration Scale
GPS	Global Positioning System
GQ-SRs	Good quality systematic reviews
HBPC	Home Based Primary Care
HDLF	Health and Daily Living Form
HDRS	Hamilton Depression Rating Scale
HSR&D	Health Services Research and Development
HTA	Health Technology Assessment
ITT	Intention-to-treat
IADL	Instrumental Activities of Daily Living scale
ICT	Information and Technology Intervention
LSIZ	Life Satisfaction Index
LSNI	Lubben Social Network Index
LTC	Long-term care
MAACL	Multiple Affect Adjective Checklist
MADDE	Medicare Alzheimer's Disease Demonstration and Evaluation program
MAI	Multilevel Assessment Inventory
MBPC	Memory and Behavior Problems Checklist

MMSE	Mini Mental State Exam
MFW	Minnesota Family Workshop
N	Number
NHS	National Health Service
NIA/NINR	National Institute on Aging/National Institute of Nursing Research
NINCDS	National Institute of Neurological and Communicative Diseases and Stroke
NPI	Neuropsychiatric Inventory
NYU	New York University
OARS	Older Americans Resource and Services Multidimensional Functional Assessment Questionnaire
OGEC	Office of Geriatrics and Extended Care
PAC	Positive Aspects of Caregiving scale
PAIS	Psychological Adjustment to Relative's Illness
PAVeD	Preventing Aggressive Behavior in Demented Patients
PCI	Patient Care Index
PDC	Partners in Dementia Care
PHQ9	Patient Health Questionnaire-9 Item
PIC	Partners in Caregiving
POMS	Profile of Moods States
QALY	Quality of adjusted life years
QOL/QoL	Quality of life
RAGE	Rating Scale for Aggressive Behavior in the Elderly
RCT	Randomized controlled trial
REACH	Resources for Enhancing Alzheimer's Caregiver Health
RIL	Record of Independent Living
RMBPC	Revised Memory and Behavior Problem Checklist
RSCSE	Revised Scale for Caregiving Self-Efficacy
SADS	Social Avoidance and Distress Scale
SBP	Stress-Busting Program
SF-36	Short-form health survey
SIP	Sickness Impact Profile
SR	Systematic Review
SSCQ	Short Sense of Competence Questionnaire
STAI	State Trait Anxiety Inventory
STAXI	State Trait Anger Expression Inventory
T1	Timepoint 1
T2	Timepoint 2
TLC	Telephone-Linked Care
Tx	Treatment
UK	United Kingdom
VA	Veterans Affairs
VAMC	Veterans Affairs Medical Center
VHA	Veterans Health Administration
VISN	Veterans Integrated Service Network
ZBI	Zarit Burden Interview

APPENDIX E. REVIEWER COMMENTS AND RESPONSES

Reviewer	Comment	Response
Question 1. Are the objectives, scope, and methods for this review clearly described?		
2	Yes. This is well written document, and the authors have done a good job of reviewing the current evidence in the field of dementia caregiver support literature – thought provoking and certainly leads to the need for a this important topic to be studied more. It will be important to identify what works to support this very burdened caregiver population.	Noted.
4	Yes. As you state, the categories are sometimes very hard to distinguish why one study is one place and not another. One particular problem I had was with the respite care section. The programs offering variety of services (p. 15, line 1) are hard to distinguish from the institutional/overnight or multi-dimensional support categories. Page 15, line 31 references basic respite care – does this refer to institutional/overnight or some other category?	We have removed the sections on multi-dimensional respite care and respite care packages that offer various forms of respite care, in order to condense the sections on respite care, and to focus on clearly defined forms of respite that are offered by or potentially feasible in VA.
	In the text descriptions of the studies, there do not appear to be consistent rules for mentioning authors (these are infrequent and when it happened, I wondered if this was a particularly good study); describing a study as small; or including the number of subjects. The number of subjects was often, but not always, listed in the text for studies pulled from the AoA compendium.	The information about studies found in the AoA compendium was derived from abstracts that did not consistently report sample size.
	One part that was missing, maybe due to the studies, is ethnic and racial diversity in caregiver interventions.	Because ethnic/racial differences were not specified in the key question, we didn't target the search strategy for literature specifically in this area. However, we did mention findings when the studies reported differential results by racial/ethnic group.
	p. 28, line 30 –One of the studies in this section did impact burden – line 13. p. 28, line 6 – comparably paced? Not sure what this means. Didn't the intervention group get data collection at the same time, too?	We have made the adjustments specified on page 28.
5	Yes. This is the most comprehensive review of caregiver stress related to dementia that I have seen. This is a sorely needed document. This document should become available for widespread use. I hope that HSR plans to produce as a booklet, much as they did for a synthesis of the literature on TBI and PTSD.	Noted.
6	Yes. The objectives and scope were outlined initially, and formed the framework of the review. This strategy was a strength of the review. I appreciated that the review was thoughtful about considering potential adverse effects of interventions, even though the literature surrounding this topic is sparse. The methods were clear as well, but required more from the reader since a full understanding of the methods required the reader to access the text, flowchart, and appendix. As I reader, I did need to interrupt the flow of my reading to understand some methodological issues that I felt were key.	Noted.

Reviewer	Comment	Response
Question 2.	**Is there any indication of bias in our synthesis of the evidence?**	
2	No. (No comment)	Noted.
5	No. This is not an issue that is a focus of commercial interests. Therefore, it is relatively easy to be free of commercial bias. I did not detect any professional bias. The process of selecting studies was fair and appropriate. The synthesis of the information was appropriate and unbiased.	Noted.
4	This isn't a methodological bias but respite care does appear to be the favored intervention, despite being the only one with reported possible negative results. (I do realize that we are already doing it, which helps.) It often has more information on it in a summary or discussion (see p. 57). For example, in the Discussion, p 51, respite is the first intervention mentioned although it is not the first one discussed in the text. I wondered if this was your ranking of the interventions.	In an effort to condense the section on respite care, we have removed sections on respite care on multi-dimensional programs and packages, and selected only clearly defined forms of respite care that are currently offered or potentially feasible in VA.
6	No. This is a very important topic to review, but also a very challenging topic. In some sense, the categorization of studies will always be arbitrary. For instance, I would not characterize a GPS intervention to prevent wandering to be similar to a tele-health (HealthBuddy) study, but these are categorized together under technology. The review notes that prior systematic reviews were not consistent in categorizing the psychosocial studies. While I did not detect bias, I think that the review could provide a stronger rationale for the way that studies were categorized for this review.	Noted. For tech-based interventions, we followed the example of a previous review that included tracking devices as well as network-based communications technology, though we agree that these interventions are dissimilar and would warrant separate categories in a review that focuses specifically on these interventions. We discuss the reasons for and challenges in grouping of interventions.
Question 3.	**Are there any studies on interventions for caregivers of patients with dementia that we have overlooked?**	
2	Not to our knowledge	Noted.
4	Yes. The behavioral studies stop in 2005 before the 2006 publication of the REACH II trial, which is indirectly cited in the two clinical translations, including the one done in VHA (REACH VA). REACH II was the largest behavioral RCT for dementia caregiving funded by NIH looking at racially and ethnically diverse caregiver. REACH is one of the evidence based programs that the Rosalynn Carter Institute for Caregiving funds. AoA has just issued another funding announcement for states to implement evidence based programs and REACH II is one of them. Funding Opportunities page on the AoA website at http://www.aoa.gov/AoARoot/ (S(olm2ek45ppxwrg45ioqbknvj))/Grants/Funding/index.aspx	We have added two studies of the REACH intervention to the section on multicomponent interventions. These studies were published more recently than the systematic reviews we had initially identified.
5	No. There are always new studies coming out. I felt that all appropriate studies within the stated collection period were included.	Noted.
6	I think that drawing from multiple past systematic reviews and the AoA catalog provides reasonable coverage. One issue that I think stands out is that there are a few caregiver interventions that enjoy such national prominence that I would have preferred the review make special mention of how they fit into the review. This happened to some extent with REACH, at least so far as the recent VA implementations of REACH are concerned. I would have appreciated some textual section that dealt with how REACH, the New York University Counseling and Support Intervention for Caregivers, and the Savvy Caregiver Program fit into the review. (Note: I am not associated with any of these, but they seem to comprise a special category at the Administration on Aging.)	Thank you for these suggestions. We have added 2 recent studies of the REACH intervention, and 1 study of the Savvy Caregiver program. The New York University Caregiver Intervention (NYUCI) was included in the initial report (Mittelman, et al.) and we have added a more recent 2007 publication of the NYUCI trial.
Question 4.	**Please write additional suggestions or comments below. If applicable, please indicate the page and line numbers from the draft report.**	

Reviewer	Comment	Response
2	Executive Summary p.vi, line 7, Individual Skills Training "CRs may benefit with slower declines in self-care when skills training includes a component targeting their activities of daily living...." It could be a consideration to suggest that individual skills training for the CR may be possible to do in the setting of the ADHC in the VA.	Agree; revised accordingly.
2	Executive Summary p. vii, line 5, Multicomponent Interventions: The outcomes are equivocal across the 2 studies, with 1 documenting differential treatment effects on an outcome of interest – time to institutionalization. Not clear what the "with 1 documenting differential treatment effects on an outcome" means? On page 45 it is clear, stating that it "significantly delayed institutionalization". Do not know if it needs to be elaborated here.	We have clarified this sentence as suggested.
2	Executive Summary, p. viii, line 12, Future Research Recommendations: The wide range of outcomes used to evaluate the effects of CG interventions reflects the diversity in what CGs and researchers consider effective. May consider using the word important for effective. I think the researchers would design interventions that they think are effective and then would measure outcomes which they think are important.	Agree; revised accordingly.
2	p.13, lines 18-19: ...problems relating to daycare attendance acted as barriers to usage for some CGs. This is a quotation from the NHS report. But it is vague what this statement means.	Agree; we have clarified by adding specific examples.
2	p. 14 lines 18-19: "There was some evidence that CRs returned home in a worse state, but also that medical conditions could be diagnosed during breaks." This is a very important point—could recommend that we should look at the VA outcomes on this from a CPRS retrospective chart review. This would help pick up the new medical conditions diagnosed, maybe not the worsening.	Agree; we have added this suggestion.
2	p. 14, line 21: "..major benefit to sleep.." Important point—not mentioned in the Executive Summary	The original Exec Summ stated, "Institutional/overnight respite promoted better sleep patterns in CGs during the period of respite..." Therefore, we have not made any changes.
2	p. 14, lines 23-24: "There was mixed evidence on the impact of services in relation to ADL, behavior and dependency, but it is difficult to unravel the potentially negative effects of respite from the natural progression of the disease." This is a quotation from the NHS report. But would it not be unlikely that a 2 week respite placement (or something like that) would impact the CR ADL, behavior and dependency due to the natural progression of the disease. It is unlikely that the disease would progress enough to impact ADL, and behavior in a short duration.	We have added this discussion point to the overnight respite care section.

Reviewer	Comment	Response
2	p. 15, lines 13-14: "A respite care model is feasible and already in place in the VA, with admission of eligible patients to skilled nursing or Community Living Center units for respite stays of approximately one week." If we have VA numbers available, may consider adding numbers here—e.g., last year there were XX respite admissions in the VA nationally. Though not all respite admissions are for patients with dementia alone.	Unfortunately I was not able to track down these figures.
2	p. 21, lines 11-16: "Another study reported no evidence that nursing case management delayed institutionalization of the CR when compared to usual care. ...Miller et al, data base reported there was no reduction in CG strain, burden, or depression resulting from nursing case management intervention that included respite care, home care, and consultation, but did find that the intervention group was more likely to use community services than the control group." Miller has reported that the intervention group was more likely to use community services than the control group. What is not known is the impact of the use of community services mentioned above.	Noted; it would be difficult to distinguish whether beneficial effects resulted from the use of community services, which was greater among those who received the nursing case management intervention (but in this case, there was no effect on CG burden). Studies specifically on the effects of the use of community services would be needed.
2	p. 21, lines 22-24: "Summary impact of case management interventions: Overall, there is little evidence to support that intensive nursing case management has a sustained impact on CG mood or strain, or on CR rates of institutionalization." The Dementia Steering Committee Report (September 2008) has recommended that there be a case manager for every dementia patient. Recommendation #44 Funding for Dementia Care Coordinators which states "VISN Leaders should allocate sufficient funds to VA facilities to ensure that veterans with dementia [have] their care coordinated through Dementia Case Managers or Care Coordinators, or Case Management teams, or CCHT teams". What do the lack of positive results using case management mean for this recommendation by the Dementia Steering Committee? Maybe the only outcome that will be positive based on the literature is more use of community resources.	Recent evidence from large, good-quality studies show significant benefit, although older studies offered little evidence to support that intensive nursing case management has a sustained impact on CG mood, strain, or rates of CR institutionalization. The 2 recent studies featured individualized assessment and care plans, and reported improvements in CG depression, stress, and confidence in caregiving, and reductions in CR problem behaviors. Although the findings are mixed across studies, there is some evidence of benefit in the most recent studies.
2	p. 48, lines 20-29: "An uncontrolled pilot study of the TLC screen program examined user satisfaction and changes in CG burden, health care utilization, and costs after 12 months." The CCHT is developing a Dementia Disease Management protocol (DMP) that is scheduled to be piloted in the next couple of months, and to be implemented nationally soon after that. It may be useful to make the recommendation that the outcomes in terms of use of technology, and other outcomes should be evaluated, maybe in a controlled trial. This has been mentioned on Page 57, line 1. But it may be helpful to add here that this should be a priority, before interventions that are not supported by the evidence go nationwide and a lot of money is spent on them.	Noted. Again, our stated purpose is to compile evidence that would help inform the decisions of policymakers. Making policy recommendations about specific interventions is beyond the scope of our report.
2	p. 53, lines 7-10: "This may indicate that the definition of what constitutes meaningful change in this field needs to be reevaluated." This is a key point. Another one is about the instruments used not being sensitive to change. While it has been mentioned in the Executive summary Page viii, lines 11-12 about the range of outcomes: "The wide range of outcomes used to evaluate the effects of CG interventions reflects the diversity in what CGs and researchers consider effective", maybe this point needs to be added to it.	Agreed. We have added the point regarding the sensitivity of instruments used.

Reviewer	Comment	Response
4	I would have loved to see you come out with a rousing endorsement of something we need to implement into VHA. As a researcher and an anthropologist, I like the idea of doing more qualitative research. As someone who knows how great the need is for caregivers, I would like to say, "Let's move forward." Maybe that is the job of the person who gets the synthesis?	Noted. We concur that the goal of this evidence review is to help inform the decisions of policymakers, although we agree that for most caregiver interventions, the results were disappointing.
4	I wondered if these articles might be of use to you in your Discussion? They are both about why we don't get findings or why our effect sizes are so small with dementia caregivers. Have you considered a composite outcome – all these studies had an effect on a component of quality of life (such as burden or depression). That would at least give us a sense of what interventions did something. Sörensen S, Pinquart M, Duberstein P. How effective are interventions with caregivers? An updated meta-analysis. Gerontologist 2002; 42: 356–372. Schulz R, Burgio L, Burns R, et al. Resources for enhancing Alzheimer's caregiver health: Overview and site specific outcomes. Gerontologist 2003; 43: 514–520.	We have added a discussion of the REACH intervention that includes Schulz 2003. We considered Sörensen 2002 in our initial review of the literature, but excluded it because the included studies were not limited to caregivers of individuals with dementia. The Sorensen 2002 analysis determined, however, that the interventions overall "were less effective at improving caregiver burden, depression, subjective well-being, and ability/knowledge when all care receivers had dementia than when care receivers did not have dementia or when the sample was mixed." This finding emphasizes that the needs of caregivers of demented individuals differ from other caregivers. Sorensen 2002 writes, "Dementia caregivers cope with unpredictable stressors, such as problem behaviors and personality changes. Because these may be more difficult to cope with and less modifiable than the stressors common to pure physical care (Birkel & Jones, 1989), it may be more difficult to effect change through intervention with this population."
4	I know it is a horrible thing to say but some people may just read the Discussion or that may be where people take major quotes from. It might make it easier for them if you spell out acronyms there, such as ICT (p. 51, line 21). I had to go back and look that one up myself!	We have added an appendix of abbreviations.
4	On pl 53, line 7, it is not clear that you are talking about all the interventions and not just respite, which leads off that paragraph.	We have clarified this sentence to read, "...among the variety of interventions for dementia caregivers."
4	For line 12, spelling out what these six important outcomes are would be helpful to the reader (not sure what they are.) Would it be helpful to include them in your methods section so that readers could be watching for the big ones as they go through?	We have clarified the outcomes referred to in that section (depression, burden, coping, quality of life, and CR behavior problems), and we list these psychosocial outcomes in the methods.
4	Discussion, p. 54, line 1 1 and Therapist may be a word that has psychological connotations to readers and may not be accurate for all the studies – perhaps interventionist? Line 12 – instrumentation issues (vary?) across sites. Line 26 – SR= systematic reviews?	We have made the suggested corrections.

Reviewer	Comment	Response
4	P. 56, recommendations. Are the studies mentioned research or clinical translations? Different connotation if they are translations – already trying to implement.	Noted. We have changed "research" to "studies" to include both types. We have also specified "feasibility of implementation" to convey the need to assess interventions that are already being implemented in VA.
5	I did not go through the document as a copy editor, so I do not have specific formatting issues to raise. My only suggestion is that this needs to be available to people outside of VHA as well as within in VHA. This may already be the plan to publish this study as an HSR&D Evidence Based Booklet. If not, I urge you to do so. This is a truly useful document.	Noted.
6	This is a valuable review that should assist policy-makers and researchers to address logical next steps. The sections describing relevance to the VA were concise and accurate.	Noted.
6	I found a fragment at the end of the sentence on line 12 pg. 54	We have made this correction.
3	In general, I found the executive summary difficult to follow and that it did not reflect the careful methods and clearer writing found in the full report.	Noted: we have revised the exec summary to provide more detail.
3	Exec Summ p. iv: "We did not assess the quality of these studies, but noted whether these more recent studies were consistent with the synthesis of findings from previous studies." Not sure what this means	We proceeded to quality-rate the studies we selected from the AoA compendium.
3	Exec Summ p. iv: "…systematic reviews that had performed comprehensive, qualitative syntheses of the primary literature on these topics." - Did you do an assessment of the quality of the reviews?	We rated the quality of systematic reviews using the criteria shown in Appendix B.
3	Exec Summ p. iv: "The systematic reviews of psychosocial interventions contained 224 primary studies, of which we identified 30 RCTs that met our criteria for study" – I would like to see a more detailed description of the number of articles that came from reviews and from other sources and how many were excluded from each, etc.	See response below (46C)
3	I am confused why you go back and forth between systematic review and the primary articles. I am used to seeing evidence based synthesis that primary use the systematic review to help find the studies to include.	Because of the sheer breadth of this topic, we conducted this primarily as a review of existing systematic reviews – we took it a step further by actually going to the primary studies (the ones we felt were best quality within the reviews we examined). The benefit of such an approach is that we can cover quite a bit of ground in a systematic way and give a "bird's eye view" of a vast/complex topic. This approach allows us to identify the types of interventions that have been studied, major gaps in the literature, and common methodologic issues in this area of study. The downside is primarily that, for any given subtopic, we are not able to do an up-to-date, complete systematic review of primary studies.
3	"significant or sustained reductions" - Are these mutually exclusive?	We have added "and/or" to indicate that these are not mutually exclusive.
3	"Three systematic reviews" - How many studies were included?	We have added the number of studies, as suggested.

Reviewer	Comment	Response
3	Exec Summ, p. v: that aimed to increase patient safety and reduce CG stress including *???*	We have made this correction.
3	Exec Summ p. vi: "Implementation of exercise interventions within the VA setting might be feasible as an outpatient group or possibly through the Home-Based Primary Care program." - These summary statements are not consistently used in each section.	We have removed the sections on feasibility from the Results sections, and added a brief section on feasibility and implementation in the Discussion.
3	Exec Summ p. vi: "Studies in which BMT for the CG was augmented by CG self-care instruction" - How many studies?	We have clarified the number of studies, as suggested.
3	Exec Summ p. vi: "The VA has provided an important training avenue for geropsychology" - Be clearer about what this means.	We have removed the statements on feasibility from most sections, and this wording was removed in the process.
3	Exec Summ p. vii: "Individualized training programs are feasible within the VA, although they would require more resources of staff to evaluate the dyad and generate a tailored program. Physical and occupational therapists and psychologists could appropriately deliver this kind of intervention." - What criteria is used to come to these conclusions? Feasibility determined by? What resources would be needed? You say that PT, OT and psychologist could deliver the interventions, but is this how they were delivered in the studies?	We have removed the sections on feasibility from the Results sections. We have added a discussion on the considerations of feasibility and implementation of interventions in VA to the Discussion section, with substantial rewording.
3	Exec Summ p. viii: "A recently completed 6-month implementation study of the REACH VA intervention found positive effects on CG burden and CR problem behaviors, and appears to be feasible and low-cost in VA settings." - I would argue that it is not truly low cost. I would argue by psychologists over multiple in home sessions.	We have removed "low-cost" from this statement, as suggested. Because individualized, resource-intensive interventions appear to be more effective, in the report we discuss the need to determine the cost-benefit of interventions that would be widely implemented in VA.
3	Exec Summ p. viii: "systematic review of respite care" - # of studies?	We have specified the number of studies, as suggested.
3	Methods, data abstraction: "and how frequently the study was included in systematic reviews." - What is the relevance of this?	The DSC had originally wondered whether there studies were widely cited but not very good evidence. We therefore sought to determine whether there were any studies that were widely known but were poor quality, and we mention this in the Discussion. We removed the data on how frequently studies were cited by other SRs from the tables, however, as we agree that this information is not obviously relevant within the tables.
3	Methods, data synthesis: We compiled a qualitative synthesis of the evidence on specific forms of therapy" - I understand what you mean by this, but I would like to know more about what went into the qualitative synthesis. Was this done by expert panel?	By this we mean that we compiled a descriptive synthesis of the evidence, as opposed to a quantitative synthesis that would combine numeric data from studies (e.g. meta-analysis). The synthesis of findings was conducted by the authors of the report, rather than the expert panel.

Interventions for Non-professional Caregivers of Individuals with Dementia

Reviewer	Comment	Response
3	Recent/ongoing research: "A 6-month feasibility study of implementing the REACH VA intervention among 24 HBPC programs in the VHA system found decreases in CG burden, depression, and time spent in caregiving; as well as decreases in CR behavior problems. REACH VA is based on the NIA/NINR funded REACH II study, and provides CG support and skills training in safety, behavior management, and self-care via 12 in-home and telephone sessions, and 5 telephone support group sessions. The analysis found that the VHA costs of delivering the full intervention would be $2.93 per day over 6 months, and that satisfaction and perception of benefit from the intervention were high among both staff and CGs." Yes, but provided to a small number of patients. Each HBPC psychologist saw a limited number of patients. It is not clear that VA current number of HBPC psychologists or other VA psychologist would have capacity to deliver this intervention to many patients.	We agree and have emphasized that although individualized, resource-intensive interventions appear to be more effective, the need to determine the cost-benefit of interventions that would be widely implemented in VA.
3	I like how the discussion is written much more than how the Executive Summary is currently written.	Noted.
1	Methods – "We also examined recently published studies, found in a compendium compiled by the Administration on Aging's Alzheimer's Disease Supportive Services Program, that were not captured in previous systematic reviews. We did not assess the quality of these studies." - Why not?	We did not formally "include" the AoA compendium because it was not a systematic review in the traditional sense, so we could not quality rate it. However, it was a very valuable resource as it has an up-to-date bibliography. Our approach was to use it as an adjunct – we looked through the compendium for more recent studies that may have had a substantial impact on the body of evidence (e.g. larger RCTs). We proceeded to quality-rate the studies we selected from the AoA for the final report.
1	Exec summary, Future research recommendations: "Respite care is already implemented in skilled care settings in the VA..." Why limit your comments to skilled care settings? VA offers respite in non-institutional settings, including home, as well as institutional (VHA Handbook 1140.02 Respite Care, Nov. 10, 2008). Respite care: "we excluded in-home respite and host-family respite care" Why exclude these? We're interested in non-institutional interventions as well as institutional. VA offers non-institutional respite care, including in-home respite services. See VHA Handbook 1140.02 Respite Care Nov. 10, 2008.	We have made this correction and have added a section on in-home respite care.
1	Wherever possible, suggest you use "individual with dementia" rather than "dementia patient"; Suggest you use "Individual with Dementia" or "Care Recipient (CR)" instead of patient	Done.
1	Page 9 –ICT interventions: Add reference for REACH study	Done.
1	p. 10 "allocation concealment" - Explain this item	We have reworded "inadequate allocation concealment" to read "potential for selection bias."
1	Respite care: "3) Respite programs – offer CGs, and CRs, a chance of combining together different forms of respite care and short breaks 4) Multi-dimensional CG-support packages – provide a range of services to CGs and CRs, including a respite or short-break option" Difference between these 2 categories is not entirely clear.	We have deleted these sections in order to condense the respite care section to represent interventions that are most applicable to VA.

Interventions for Non-professional Caregivers of Individuals with Dementia

Reviewer	Comment	Response
1	Respite care, Page 14: Overall, a day treatment model is feasible within the VA, and is currently deployed in individual VA settings with other populations (e.g. substance abuse treatment, chronically mentally ill). We did not find a VA-specific utilization/cost report for dementia day care, but community hospital programs have demonstrated cost savings through dementia day care programs.14 Are you including VA's Adult Day Health Care in this discussion of "day treatment model"? Seems like it should be mentioned. See VHA Handbook 1141.03 Adult Day Health Care, Sept. 29, 2009. There was a VA HSR&D evaluation of the ADHC program in the distant past, I believe – not dementia-specific, but of the program as a whole.	We have removed the feasibility statements from the Results section and in the process, the text cited was deleted.
1	Respite Care – Institutional/overnight Services "This model appears suitable for a VA setting , " This is already an option in VA.	We have made this correction.
1	"Respite Care – Programs Offering a Variety of Respite Services and Short Breaks" Not entirely clear how this group differs from those in the next section.	We have added a description of the multi-dimensional CG support packages that distinguishes those interventions from respite services alone.
1	"Respite programs provide a variety of forms of respite to accommodate the needs and preferences of the CG and CR." Can you describe the range of services/studies a little more? Not sure what this group actually includes.	We have added a description of the different respite programs offered in the included studies.
1	"A respite care model is feasible and already in place in the VA, with admission of eligible patients to skilled nursing or Community Living Center units for respite stays of approximately one week." VA CLCs are skilled nursing, so "or" seems wrong here; can you clarify meaning or wording?	We have removed the sections on feasibility from the Results sections and in the process, this sentence was eliminated.
1	"Respite Care – Multi-dimensional CG Support Packages The NHS report identified 4 studies in which a range of services was provided, including a respite or short-break option." Can you describe the range of services/studies a little more? Not sure what this group actually includes.	We have added the description of the range of services provided by the NHS report.
1	Respite Care – Multi-dimensional CG Support Packages: "This program would require more specialized resources within the VA system, and does not appear to have a clear advantage in long-term outcome over basic respite care." What do you mean by "this program"? You have not described a specific program.	We have deleted this section and condensed the respite care section to represent interventions that are most applicable to VA.
1	"Psychosocial Interventions – Exercise Training: Two studies evaluated exercise training (Table 1). In one study, CGs participated in an exercise training program that successfully cultivated adherence to regular exercise participation" Is this exercise by CR or CG?	We have clarified this, as suggested, in the tables and text.
1	Psychosocial Interventions – Case Management: Can you take a look at the following two studies and see if they fit this or one of the other categories of studies you are reviewing? These are multi-component care management models that may have effects on CG and CR. Callahan, Boustani, et al., 2006, JAMA 295(18),2148-57. Vickrey et al., 2006, Ann Intern Med 145:713-26.	We have added the suggested studies to the case management section.

Reviewer	Comment	Response
1	Table 3: There are CG outcome measures, so aren't there CG results to report?	We have clarified the tables to indicate whether CG (or CR) outcomes were measured as covariates only or analyzed as outcomes of the intervention.
1	Discussion: p.56 "Future studies should use … adequate duration of follow-up" – Did you mention this earlier as a limitation?	We have changed "adequate" to "appropriate" duration of follow-up, given that benefit from some interventions may be short-term.
1	last paragraph of discussion (before references): "supportive" – Clarify what you mean by this term. Is it all other intervention types examined in this review, or just some types?	We have removed the term "supportive" to convey that we are referring to all CG interventions.
1	"Our informal survey of recently completed and ongoing research using VA e-mail listservs identified preliminary studies of psychosocial interventions (REACH OUT57; REACH VA56; Stress-Buster's Program62) and technology-based interventions (Telehealth Education Program60; TLC58) that found improvements in CG burden with some of the interventions, and short-term savings in health care costs in one study ." Add reference citation number (for last study)	Done.
1	Future research recommendations: In this section or somewhere else in the Discussion – Do you think any of the specific interventions that we don't already provide are ready for wide-spread roll-out/implementation in VA?	It appears that the salient feature in effective interventions is the individualized assessment and construction of interventions that are tailored to the needs of the dyad. Multicomponent interventions appear to be more effective than single-intervention approaches. We have added this to the Discussion.
1	Future research recommendationsAt the end of this section, are there any more specific research recommendations to make? This final section seems almost all about respite.	We have removed some of the text in this section to de-emphasize respite care.
1	Discussion: "We attempted to examine the performance of measures for CG depression, burden, and CR behavior problems across the 30 studies reviewed here, but the samples were too small to derive strong conclusions about the hit rates of the measures." - Clarify term (hit rates)	We have replaced "hit rates of the measures" with "whether specific measures were more likely to detect improvements".
1	Discussion: "global ratings of distress and burden may not reflect the changes or possible benefits that CGs may be experiencing. Yet these measures continue to be used widely." - What is an alternative that should be used instead?	We discuss in Future Research Recommendations the need to develop/identify alternative measures to gauge the effectiveness of CG interventions, given the complexity in the needs of CGs.
1	"we did not proceed to search for recently published RCTs ." I don't understand this reasoning. I think you should search for more recent ones!	We agree and have quality-rated the studies we selected from the AoA compendium.